PRAISE FOR ANI PHYO:

"*Not* cooking can take as much time as cooking, but this guide to goin
   —*New York Times*

"The raw-food stylings of the uncook queen Ani Phyo return for her most must-have volume yet. *Ani's Raw Food Essentials* hits all of the basics—and beyond—in its hefty 300+ pages. Written with the beginner in mind, Phyo's comprehensive content makes it perfect for anyone interested in adding more raw, unprocessed, delicious, and healthy meals to their life . . . Phyo's tone is nothing but positive and supportive, encouraging small steps toward a healthier lifestyle and never demanding a 100-percent raw diet—especially not overnight."
   —*VegNews*

"Phyo . . . is one of the leaders of raw food's latest cycle, thanks to the clever, uncomplicated recipes she develops . . . [her] desserts are universally appealing."
   —*Food & Wine*

"Phyo's book proves that raw foods are not only easy to make, but also tasty."
   —*Arizona Republic*

"Ani's food is . . . inspiring. This book . . . makes raw cuisine accessible for everyone to enjoy."
   —*Juliano Brotman, author of* Raw, the Uncook Book

"Her array of delicious recipes will convince you that eating raw is not impossible and definitely not boring."
   —*Curve*

"*Ani's Raw Food Kitchen* will surprise you with recipes that somehow seem very familiar even if you've never eaten them before. [H]er advice is easy to implement and her recipes are often quick to prepare."
   —boingboing.net

"Reading *Ani's Raw Food Kitchen* is a must if you want to treat your body with first-class nutrition and your mind with first-class advice. Reading and following Ani's directions is time well spent."
   —Howard Lyman (the Mad Cowboy)

"As someone who has just recently discovered raw food and all its glory Ani's books and recipes have been both inspiring and exciting. The recipes I've made have been delicious and impressed even my non–raw food friends."
   —Carrie-Anne Moss, Actress

ani's
RAW FOOD
asia

EASY EAST-WEST FUSION RECIPES

Ani Phyo

Da Capo
LIFE
LONG

A Member of the Perseus Books Group

I dedicate this book to my mother, in loving memory to my late father, and to my brother for blessing me with a healthy, happy, privileged life that's infused with the best of everything from the East and the West.

Photography and illustrations by:

Tyler Golden (recipe photographs, pages 16, 24–25, 28–29, 32, 67, 71, 75, 80, 90, 94, 96–97, 100–101, 112, 115, 116, 122, 138, 164, 172, 181, 183, 198, 204, 211, 213, 223, 224–225, 232, 249, 251, 253, 260–216)

Anthony Hall (Asia photographs, pages 1–3, 6, 8, 34–35, 42–43, 62–63, 86, 95, 102–103, 126–127, 132, 154–155, 159, 185, 205, 214–215, 240–241, 255, 268–269, 276–277)

Arthur Davis III & Maria Loewenstein as KingVictoria™ (Ani in Asia photographs, pages 64, 104–105, 121)

Marieke Derks (Ani in Asian Kitchen photographs, pages 219 & 279)

Carol Conforti (pages 48 & 246)

Antonio Sanchez (icon illustrations)

All other photos by Ani Phyo

Designed by Megan Jones Design (www.meganjonesdesign.com)
Set in 10 point Chaparral Pro by Megan Jones Design (www.meganjonesdesign.com)

Cataloging-in-Publication data for this book is available from the Library of Congress.

First Da Capo Press edition 2011
ISBN: 978-0-7382-1457-3

Published by Da Capo Press
A Member of the Perseus Books Group
www.dacapopress.com

Note: The information in this book is true and complete to the best of our knowledge. This book is intended only as an informative guide for those wishing to know more about health issues. In no way is this book intended to replace, countermand, or conflict with the advice given to you by your own physician. The ultimate decision concerning care should be made between you and your doctor. We strongly recommend you follow his or her advice. Information in this book is general and is offered with no guarantees on the part of the authors or Da Capo Press. The authors and publisher disclaim all liability in connection with the use of this book. The names and identifying details of people associated with events described in this book have been changed. Any similarity to actual persons is coincidental.

Da Capo Press books are available at special discounts for bulk purchases in the U.S. by corporations, institutions, and other organizations. For more information, please contact the Special Markets Department at the Perseus Books Group, 2300 Chestnut Street, Suite 200, Philadelphia, PA, 19103, or call (800) 810–4145, ext. 5000, or e-mail special.markets@perseusbooks.com.

10 9 8 7 6 5 4 3 2 1

contents

2   salads and dressings   59

3 pickles, condiments, and accompaniments 81

6 rolls, wraps, and pancakes   155

7   noodles   193

8 rice 215

9 desserts 241

10 menus 269

afterword: RAW FOOD FOR LONGEVITY   277

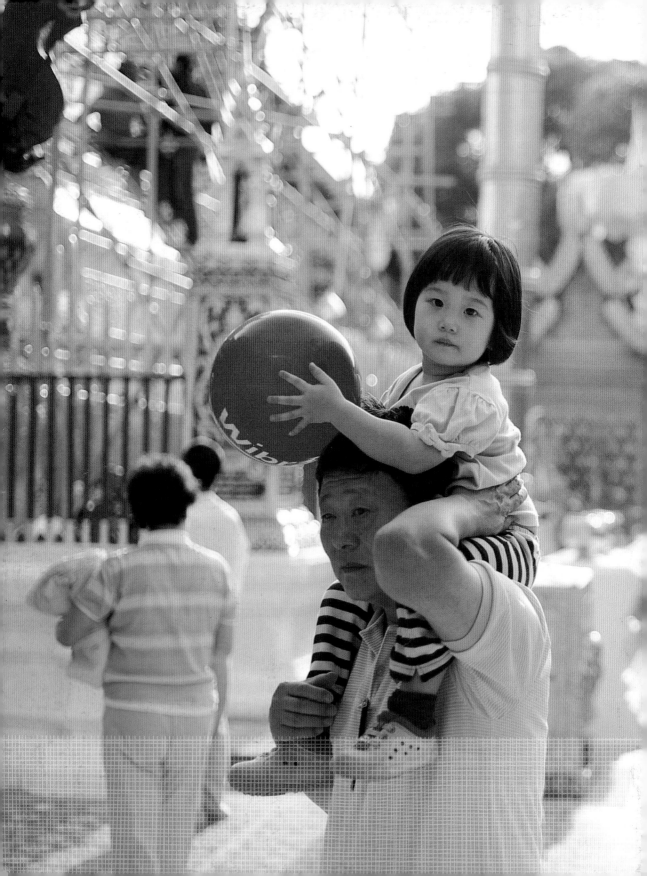

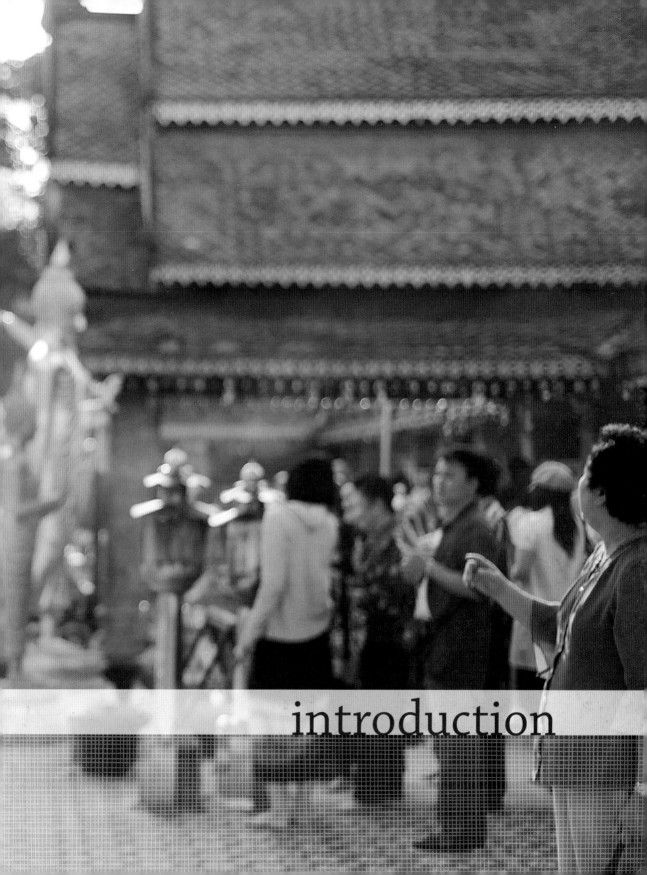

introduction

Growing Up Korean American

I'm the daughter of two Korean immigrants; North and South Korean culture were both a part of our home. Our Korean language, food, and lifestyle were all very different from the culturally diverse American world outside our doors. We lived an eco green lifestyle in an eco home, and my parents were the first raw fooders and green lifestylists I ever knew.

Some of my earliest memories are of our home in Nashville, Tennessee, when I was four. I remember the warm sun, snipping the top of my little brother's head bald while playing barbershop, and making mud pies that didn't taste so good. I worried my Mom sick once by disappearing; she later found me at the home of my Indian neighbor. Mrs. Rao had found me lingering outside her front door and invited me in to feed me her delicious home-cooked Indian food. To this day, the rich, complex flavors of Indian food are still some of my favorites.

The rest of my youth was spent in smaller rural and suburban communities that were pretty much all Caucasian. As with most Korean first-generation children, I was encouraged to study and work hard and to practice playing piano and violin, and I was required to study Korean by reading from a stack of workbooks every Saturday morning. All I wanted to do was to watch Saturday morning cartoons. I missed out on that and wasn't allowed to watch much television at all.

The glimpses of television I caught reflected what I had thought was the real-world America, out there. For many years, I denied my Asian heritage in an attempt to be more "American." I wanted to fit in, and for a brief time, even tricked myself into thinking I was Caucasian, only to be reminded I looked different by the occasional intentional, and unintentional, racist comment.

I've spent my adult years living in ethnically diverse, large metropolitan cities: New York City, London, Sydney, San Francisco, and Los Angeles. Each boasts its own Chinatown, Little India, Thai Town, Koreatown, and Little Tokyo, to name a few. These cities embrace the multiculturalism that makes up our real America. A recent trip to Southeast Asia made me realize that our real-world America is not reflected in our homogenous, mainstream media.

The mainstream American media propagates an unhealthy Caucasian American image of meat and potatoes, cholesterol-laden dishes, deep-fried foods, white flour, sugar, and processed and fast foods. This is our Standard American Diet—known by the telling acronym SAD. By eating processed food prepared with fat, sugar, and cholesterol, many Americans also end up looking like the unhealthy, overweight television cooking show hosts who are teaching us how to prepare these dishes. On the flip side, air-brushed and plastic surgery–"enhanced" images of unattainable and unnatural beauty have helped to cause anorexia in a friend's ten-year-old daughter. Our media sells us fad weight-loss programs, diet pills, and quick fixes—at the same time it promotes an unhealthy cuisine and lifestyle.

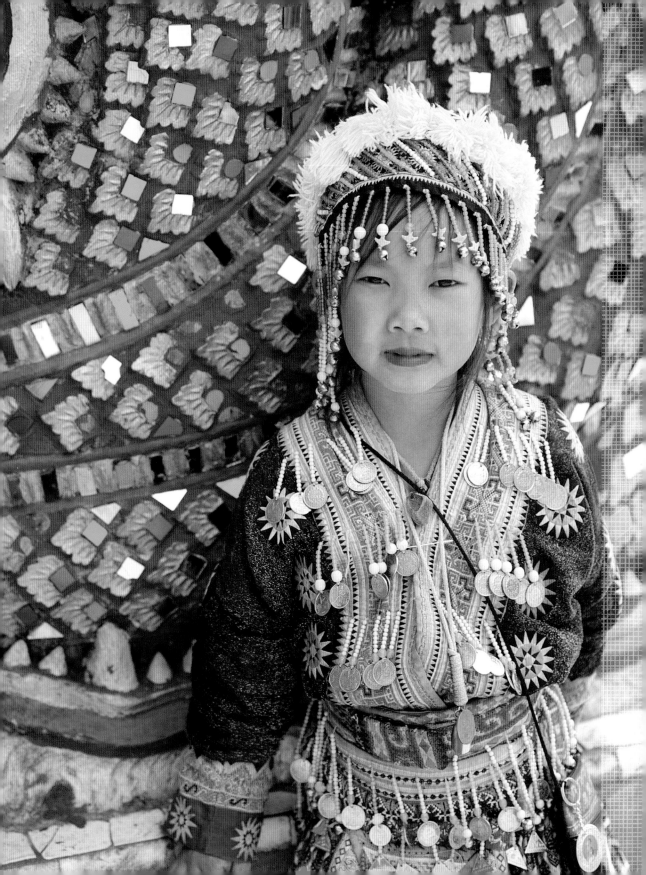

The American media is slowly changing, and we're starting to see programming designed to help teach people how to live healthy, active, and happy lives. I hope to see more positive programming that encourages us to strive for vitality and strength through exercise, nutrition, rest, community, and happiness instead of vanity-driven weight loss or weight gain via processed supplements, powders, and pills. It would become fashionable to be vibrant and healthy, glowing from the inside out with radiant skin and a clear complexion. We're starting to pay more attention to our resources, environment, food, water, health of our animals, and well-being of humans as being connected together as one living organism. This is the way it's been for thousands of years in Asian culture.

Today, I am finally proud to be a Korean American. Perhaps it's partially due to the fact Asia has now come into fashion. We Westerners look to the East for yoga, meditation, spirituality, and religion; Chinese and Ayurvedic medicine, and acupuncture; and ancient beauty, weight-loss, and longevity secrets. We look to Asia for the keys of living life well to prevent, rather than to mask, symptoms of illness and disease.

I hope to help bridge the gap between the "steak-and-potatoes America" propagated by our media with the Asian eco-lifestyle and diet that's part of my heritage and culture. I'm excited to share with you my unique style of Raw Asian American Fusion Cuisine that will bring everyone one step closer along our journeys to ultimate health, vitality, beauty, happiness, well-being, and living a long and prosperous Super Life.

In addition to my Asian-inspired recipes, I share my take on wellness, fitness, eco-green clean living, entertaining, happiness, and things I do to live a life that's super. I hope you'll join me. Go Super Life!

SMARTMONKEY FOODS

In Chinese astrology, I was born in the year of the monkey, and my dad's nickname for me was always SmartMonkey. I thought this name was perfect as the name of my first raw food business, SmartMonkey Foods, since raw foods are eaten by the smartest monkeys on the planet.

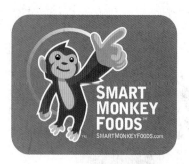

Fresh, Living Cuisine

By enjoying raw foods, I get to eat the wide variety of delicious and nutritious fresh and whole fruits, vegetables, nuts, and seeds in Mother Nature's bounty. I strive to place the lowest impact on our planet Earth and on my body, so my raw foods are organic, local, and seasonal whenever possible. Geography and climate will affect the availability of fresh local produce, so I will try to do the best I can while keeping my lifestyle, environment, and climate in mind. No one is perfect, and for me, striving for perfection is too stressful.

My belief is that everyone benefits from introducing more fresh produce into any diet. I prefer to eat most of my food fresh, though sometimes they may be dehydrated, or dried, at low temperatures. I've even been known to heat up a soup or chili that's come out of the cold fridge on my stove. But, my ingredients are usually not heated above 104°F, and rarely cooked.

Heat damages beneficial vitamins, minerals, amino acids, and enzymes in fresh food. While lowering the nutritional value of our food, heating also releases water. Our bodies are made up of about 80 percent water, and so is the planet. Most people are under-hydrated, so I like to ingest my water through the foods I eat as much as possible. Plants naturally distill water, and by eating water-rich plant-based foods, we're eating living water rather than dead water that's been sitting stagnant inside a toxic plastic bottle.

My approach to raw foods focuses on health, vitality, and longevity. Raw food is perfect for detoxing and cleansing, hands down. It's great for boosting immunity, helping our bodies achieve their ideal weight, clearing up our skin and allergies, and for treading lightly on our planet. I hope to help people live better lives through better nutrition because when we are healthy, strong, vibrant, and feel good in our body, it's easy to be happy. And, from this place, achieving any goal is possible.

I encourage you to find what works for you. Choose your own path. No one outside of yourself will be able to tell you what to do. What works for one person will not work for another. There's never just one answer that works for everyone. We all have unique bodies and come from different cultural backgrounds, ethnicities, and histories.

Whether you're coming to raw foods from a Standard American Diet of dairy and meat, a vegan diet, or a vegetarian diet, I believe adding more fresh raw foods will make you healthier, stronger, lighter, and happier. If you're eating meat, consider thinking of it more as a side dish or accompaniment, rather than the main, as it is in Asia. Add my recipes to any meal as additional sides and main dishes for a fresher twist.

After each meal, take note of how you feel. Chances are that after a meal that includes more fresh, whole, raw foods you'll feel lighter, more energetic, and stronger. You'll probably find you can think more clearly, are able to focus better, and are more productive. All this may make you feel better about yourself, and the hop in your step will make you look your best, too.

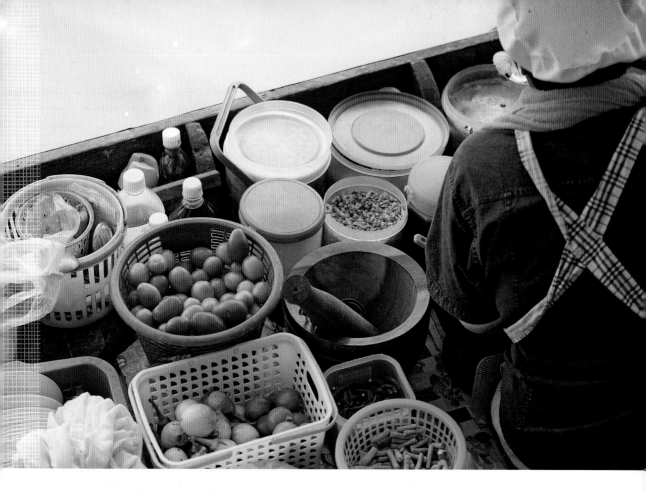

THREE STYLES OF ASIAN CUISINE

Asian food blends together sweet, sour, salty, spicy, and bitter while emphasizing a combination of flavors, textures, and colors within a single dish. Asian cooks, especially in the southern regions, prepare spice blends by freshly blending or grinding whole spices and preparing curry mixes. Anthropologists identify three categories, based on culture, of Asian dietary styles: the southwest, the northeast, and the southeast.

Southwest Asian countries include India, Pakistan, Sri Lanka, and Burma. Their roots are in Persian-Arabian civilization, and spices used include chile pepper, black pepper, cloves, cinnamon, coriander, cumin, nutmeg, cardamom, ginger, mustard, and turmeric. Hinduism is prevalent in these cultures, and cows are not eaten for meat.

>>>

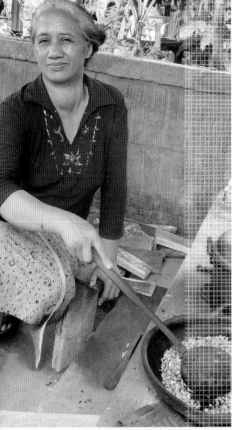

>>>

The northeast region includes Korea, China, and Japan, where oils and sauces are used in cooking. Foods, spices, and seasonings are used as medicines to promote a long and healthy life, and people use food as symbolic offerings when worshiping their ancestors. These cultures are influenced by Buddhism, and traditionally adhere to vegetarianism.

Korean food uses red chiles, ginger, soybean paste (miso), soy sauce, toasted sesame oil, sea vegetables, and pickled vegetables to make varieties of probiotic kimchis. Southern Chinese food emphasizes freshness, while Northern Chinese cuisine uses more vinegar and garlic with oil due to the colder climate. Japanese food is simple and fresh, with some deep-frying, as in tempura, and uses sea vegetables.

The southeast includes Thailand, Laos, Cambodia, Vietnam, Indonesia, Malaysia, Singapore, and Brunei. Emphasis is on aromatic, lightly prepared foods with spices and seasonings, including basil, cilantro, Asian lime leaf (aka Kaffir lime), lemongrass, Thai basil, lemon basil, Vietnamese mint, black sesame seed, coconut, galangal, and star anise. Religious influences include Buddhist, Hindu, and Islam.

The recipes in this book are my own unique style of Asian American fusion. They are inspired by the flavors from southwest, northeast, and southeast Asia and are not designed to mimic or replace traditional Asian cooked dishes. My recipes are designed to stand alone with their own full flavor profiles as delicious, beautiful, and healthy cuisine for fueling a long and Super Life.

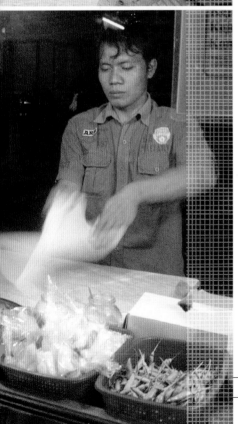

Raw Food: More Than Just a Diet

Raw food is a lifestyle taking us back to eating the way our grandparents did, before the industrialization of our food. Through raw, whole, fresh foods, we connect directly to our food source . . . the earth, our community, and our local farmers. So much of our food today is processed: denatured and manufactured by machines in a factory. And, our children don't understand what real food is, let alone where it comes from.

Natural food grocery chains and co-ops have become more popular and mainstream. So has the popularity of organic, local, and seasonal foods. A silver lining that's come out of our recent hard-hit economic times is that more people now make food at home. Many have started to grow their food in a home or community garden, and farmers' markets are popping up everywhere.

With the growing obesity epidemic, along with the rise of health issues like heart disease, diabetes, and cancer, people are starting to understand the connection between health and food choices. Now more than ever, people are interested in preventative care to offset expensive medical bills later.

Raw foods help increase vitality and slow down our aging process. Raw foods strengthen our immune system, helps us lose unwanted extra pounds, and offer the ultimate for detoxing, cleansing, and rebuilding our bodies. One-hundred percent natural without chemicals or manufactured or processed ingredients; raw foods have been shown to reverse serious health conditions and are great to enjoy every day to prevent sickness and maintain health.

WHOLE FOOD NUTRITION

Fruits, vegetables, nuts, and seeds are touted as "superfoods" by the U.S. Food and Drug Administration (FDA) because they are high in antioxidants, vitamins, minerals, and amino acids. They help combat free-radical damage, slow down the signs of aging, and provide our skin with nutrients that build collagen and keep us looking younger, longer. They fuel our bodies with the building blocks we need to recover after a stressful day, and to regenerate a stronger, leaner, and more vibrant body.

As gifts from Mother Nature, these superfood ingredients are recognizable to our body, and take less energy to break down, digest, absorb, and then eliminate. We don't have to work as hard to fuel ourselves, decreasing wear and tear on our digestive system and overall stress on our body.

WATER AND FIBER

Fresh whole foods provide naturally distilled and structured water. The plant pulls mineral-rich water from the Earth's soil up through its roots, in turn distilling it and providing us with living water. A natural way to hydrate is by eating fresh fruits and vegetables.

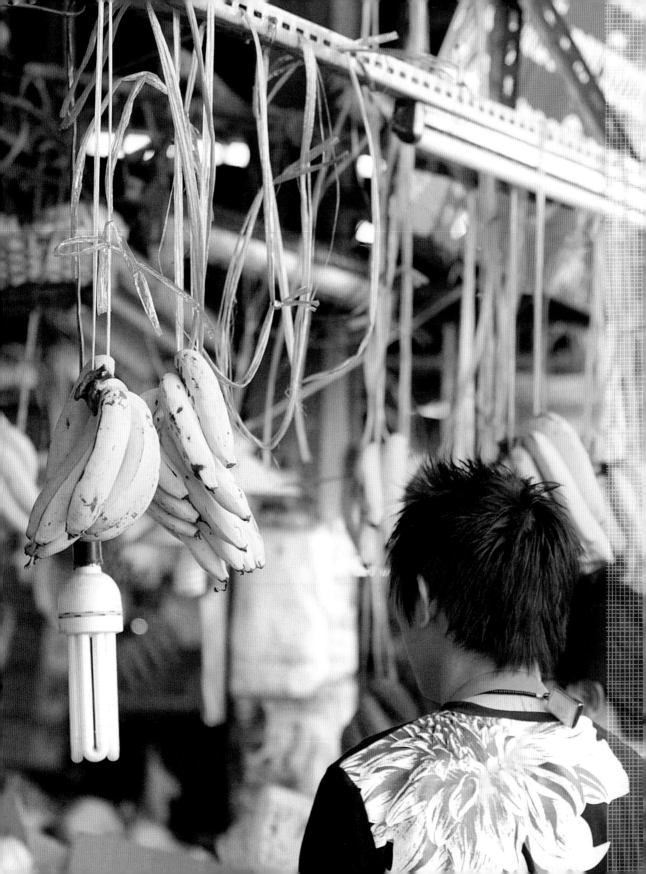

Fruits, vegetables, nuts, and seeds are packed with fiber, which acts like a broom sweeping our insides clean. The water is like a hose washing us out. Raw foods help us practice personal hygiene from the inside out. It's naturally cleansing and detoxifying.

LOCAL AND SEASONAL

I prefer shopping locally and seasonally whenever possible. Seasonal foods are at their peak for flavor and nutritional value so I get more for my money. Shopping locally means I'm decreasing energy used to transport and warehouse food from far-away places. I'm able to buy fresh produce that's been picked a few hours prior and brought to me at my local farmers' market, which means it lasts longer in my fridge, Plus, I get to keep my money within my community to support my local farmer friends.

FOOD SAFETY

By going straight to the source for my fresh, whole foods, there are fewer places along the way where manufacturers can sneak in some toxic chemical coloring, flavoring, preservative, pesticide, herbicide, or other unwanted poison into what I eat. Touch points where bacteria and other contaminants can be introduced are decreased to keep my food cleaner . . . and safer.

Kitchen Tools and Techniques

Setting up a raw kitchen is easy. The first step is making sure you have the right tools, and the two I like to start everyone out with are a food processor, which you can find for around $50, and a high-speed blender, which costs a few hundred dollars. If you want to acquire equipment in stages, start with the food processor and a smaller blender/grinder called the Personal Blender.

BLENDING VS. PROCESSING

The blender is used to whip up ingredients with water to create a kream or pudding with a smooth texture, and a drink like a shake and mylk. The food processor, on the other hand, is for chopping up dry or whole ingredients, without adding more additional liquids.

 FOOD PROCESSOR

A food processor will save you hours of chopping time. It processes and chops into small bits nuts, seeds, vegetables, and fruits. It usually comes with attachments for shredding and slicing, too.

HIGH-SPEED BLENDER

The blender I've been using forever is the Vitamix. I've used it to make food for thousands and thousands of people over the years, and it keeps going strong. A Vitamix costs about $500, but it will outlast five $100 blenders, I promise. Look for the model with the variable speed dial in the center, rather than just the on/off and high/low switches to avoid splattering of your sauce all over the inside of the container. I have an additional 4-cup wet container, as well as the larger 8-cup, and recommend considering adding a dry blade container for grinding larger quantities of dry ingredients. The Vita-Prep Commerical Food Prep Blender is about $500, and is available at www.GoSuperLife.com.

PERSONAL BLENDER

This mini-blender is my favorite for making single- or double-serving smoothies, sauces, and dressings. I like to bring it with me when I travel, as it takes up very little room in my luggage. The Personal Blender comes with a blender top and also a grinder top for grinding nuts and seeds into a powder. It comes with lids so you can make your sauce and store it all in the same container to decrease cleanup and extra dishes to wash. It also comes with a commuter lid so you can blend and take it with you when you run out the door in the morning. If you're just putting together your raw kitchen, you may want to start with the Personal Blender first, upgrading to a Vitamix at a later date. The Personal Blender costs about $100 and is available at www.GoSuperLife.com.

SUN BAKING

In a raw food kitchen, a dehydrator is our oven. A dehydrator is a sun-drying simulator that allows us to dry our food at low temperatures. Dehydrators come in a box shape with shelves that sit inside or in a stackable tray design. The stackable tray dehydrators cost less and are flexible to grow and shrink by adding or removing trays to accommodate your batch size. However, they have a channel up the center for airflow, which means the trays have a cut-out circle in the center. So, you can't make a 14 by 14-inch square of crepe or cracker. But the lower-priced stackable makes it a great place to start. You can always invest in the larger box-shaped Excalibur later.

DEHYDRATOR

I love my Excalibur nine-tray with built-in timer, which costs about $199 at www.GoSuper Life.com. I recommend purchasing reusable ParaFlexx non-stick sheets for your Excalibur.

GRINDING

For some raw food recipes, you'll need to make powders from whole seeds and nuts. You can do this with your Vitamix dry container, if you have one. I avoid using my wet container to grind because it dulls my blades. Nuts can be ground in a food processor to make a flour or meal. But for small seeds, like sesame or flax, it's best to use a coffee grinder. Or, use the grinding lid that comes with your Personal Blender.

RETRO COFFEE GRINDER

The Personal Blender comes with a grinder attachment that works great, or you can use a coffee grinder.

MORTAR AND PESTLE

A mortar and pestle is used to crush, grind, and hand pound aromatics into a flavorful paste. Choose one that's made of a strong material that won't break under pressure, like granite. Avoid brittle lava rock that can result in gritty pastes and chipped teeth. The cavity should be deep and wide enough to hold all your ingredients in the bottom one-third. A stone mortar and pestle becomes well seasoned over time, so you never want to wash it with soap, just water. To remove an aromatic characteristic out of your mortar and pestle, just pound some raw rice in it to absorb oils and flavors, then rinse with water.

STRAINING

I have strainers of several sizes in my kitchen, some in metal mesh and some in plastic mesh.

COLANDER

A large colander is good to have for draining kelp noodles and greens.

STRAINING SIEVE

A smaller, finer strainer is good for straining seeds and nuts when soaking and/or sprouting.

NUT MYLK BAG, AKA FILTERING BAG

A filtering bag is made of a cheesecloth type material to help strain the liquid while trapping in the fiber for a smoother, lighter milk texture. I personally like the fiber in my drinks and don't usually use nut mylk bags. But they may be fun to have if you prefer straining your mylks for a smoother texture.

JUICING

Citrus juicers make juicing lemons and limes easier, and they come in hand-operated and motorized electric versions.

CITRUS JUICER
For home use, I find a hand juicer to work fine for extracting the juice from my lemons and limes.

VEGETABLE JUICER
Vegetable juicers are great to have in any kitchen to make mineral rich green juices. You can find one starting from about 50 to 75 dollars. I recommend choosing one that has a large opening that will fit a whole apple or lemon, and catches all the pulp in one place so that it's easy to clean. The recipes in this book don't require a vegetable juicer, but they're still nice to have.

ESSENTIALS

Every kitchen needs essentials like measuring spoons and cups, mixing bowls, and knives. Mason jars are great for pickling, but also for storing herbs, nuts, seeds, sauces, and mylks. I keep plastic gloves on hand for when I need to massage hot peppers into my recipe, or just feel like avoiding getting sticky ingredients all over my hands.

KNIFE
I have a mix of different sizes, shapes, and styles. I like my razor sharp stainless steel Global from Japan, but I love my ceramic knives best. Ceramic doesn't need sharpening, ever. Plus, it keeps my food fresher longer than the oxidizing reaction of a metal blade. Ceramic knives are available at www.GoSuperLife.com.

MASON JAR
Every raw kitchen needs glass jars. They can be purchased mason jars, or reused glass jars from almond butter. Use them to store nuts, seeds, spices, and spirulina powder. Use 1-quart glass jars for pickling.

GLOVES
It's not environmentally friendly to use disposable gloves made of latex or plastic, but they're handy to have in the kitchen. Wearing gloves when mixing together spicy kimchi will keep your hands from burning up.

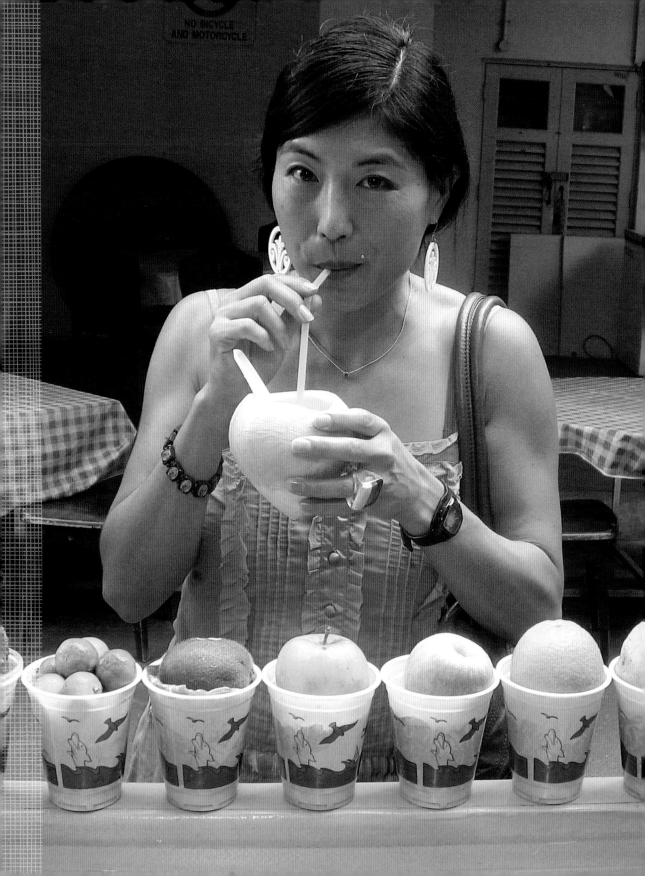

FUN TO HAVE

The following tools make playtime in the kitchen more fun. Having the right tools speeds up prep time and makes creating shapes and textures easier. If you don't have these, you can find work-arounds, but consider adding these to your toolkit over time.

MICRO PLANER

A micro planer is great for zesting and grating garlic, nutmeg, and ginger.

MANDOLINE SLICER

Helps you slice paper thin, even pieces of fruits and vegetables. You can always slice by hand if needed.

SPIRALIZER

This tool will help you slice angel hair shaped "noodles" with vegetables like zucchini, beets, and carrots. You can always slice noodles by hand if needed.

ICE CREAM MAKER

Pour in your nut kream and watch it firm up and freeze in an ice cream maker. Nice to have, but you can always just freeze your batter in a container in the freezer overnight instead.

ICE CREAM SCOOPER

Scoopers are great for more than just ice cream. They're good for portioning batter and shaping cookies.

CHOCOLATE MOULD TRAY

Will make pretty shapes for Sweet Sesame Halvah candies and chocolates. Ice cube trays work, too.

COCKTAIL SHAKER

Shakers and strainers are fun for cocktail parties. Large pint glasses and a straining sieve will work, too.

WHISK

Helpful in mixing together sauces, but you can always use a fork.

TIPS

The icons below help signal these tips.

 If it's cold out, if you don't care to eat cold food straight out of the fridge, or if you're just craving something warm, go ahead and warm up my raw food recipes in a saucepan or oven. These recipes are made from whole food ingredients with no fillers, chemicals, preservatives, artificial colorings, or flavors. While enzymes and nutritional value are damaged by the higher heat we apply to cook, what's important to remember is that this food is still clean, free of allergens like wheat, soy, and dairy, and is good for your health. If heating will help you get more whole food, local, organic, natural ingredients into your diet, then go for it. Flexibility, moderation, gratitude, and happiness are keys to longevity.

 My tips for longevity to help you Go Super Life!

 Eco green living tips that help us tread lighter on the planet.

 Fun tidbits and ideas.

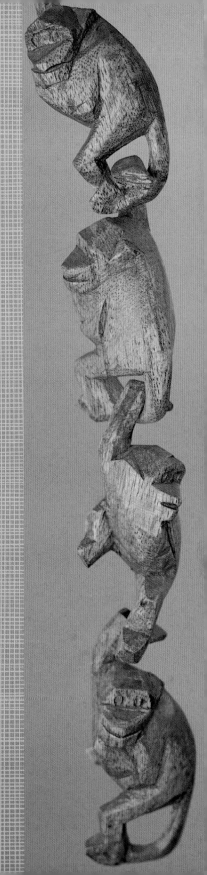

Ingredients and Substitutions

I've designed the recipes in this book to use easy-to-find, everyday ingredients. For some harder-to-find ingredients, like galangal root, I replace with ginger. Most can be found at your local farmers' market or local natural food store.

I couldn't resist including a couple of my favorite recipes that use harder-to-find Asian fruits like durian, jackfruit, and lychee, but I do offer substitutions in the recipe itself for these ingredients.

ASIAN AISLE

These ingredients are typically found in the Asian isle of most mainstream groceries, and are available at natural food stores. Most of the following Asian ingredients are available online at: www.GoSuperLife.com.

SEA VEGETABLES

A great source for protein, iodine, and minerals. See the sidebar Ancient Longevity Secret: Seaweed (page 140).

- Arame
- Dulse
- Wakame
- Nori

KOREAN CHILE POWDER AND FLAKES

Nice to have if available. Or, substitute with cayenne and red chile flakes to taste. Korean chile powder is milder.

NAMA SHOYU

A raw, unpasteurized soy sauce. Substitute with Bragg Liquid Aminos, tamari, or soy sauce.

BRAGG LIQUID AMINOS

Gluten-free soy sauce substitute, is considered a living food with enzymes. Substitute with tamari.

TAMARI

Cooked gluten-free soy sauce. Substitute with Bragg Liquid Aminos.

GOJI BERRIES

A dry, sweet, red berry with many health benefits. See the sidebar Goji Berries for Longevity (page 265). Can be substituted with dried berries, cherries, or raisins in recipes.

DRY SHIITAKE MUSHROOMS

Korean homes always keep dried mushrooms on hand. They are easily rehydrated. I always prefer fresh, but it's nice to keep some dried ones in the pantry, too.

PRODUCE

The following are fresh Asian ingredients found in most supermarket produce departments. Always choose organic when possible.

SHIITAKE MUSHROOMS

These have a distinct Asian flavor. Can be substituted with any mushroom.

FRESH THAI RED CHILES

A spicy hot chile. Can be substituted with any fresh chile such as jalapeño.

SCALLION OR GREEN ONION

Two names for the same long spring onion.

SHALLOTS

Tastes like an onion, but sweeter and milder in flavor. You can substitute with sweet onion.

LEMONGRASS

Comes in long stalks and has a lemony scent. Has refreshing, light flavor with a hint of ginger.

THAI YOUNG COCONUT

White and shaved down with a point at the top. Here in the States, the coconuts are wrapped in plastic. Different from the hairy brown coconuts.

JICAMA

A crispy, light, sweet-tasting root that looks like a grapefruit-size round turnip. Cultivated in Asia and also South America and popular in South Asian as well as Mexican cuisine.

DAIKON RADISH

A large, white, East Asian radish that's mild in flavor and shaped like a big carrot. Can be substituted with jicama.

MUNG BEAN SPROUTS

Large white sprouts with thick stalks that are juicy and crisp. Substitute with another large sprout like sunflower sprouts, or wispy alfalfa or broccoli sprouts.

ASIAN LIME LEAF

The Asian lime is a bumpy-skinned green fruit whose leaves are aromatic and shaped in double leaves. Often called Kaffir lime, I recently discovered "kaffir" is a derogatory term used toward Africans, and the politically correct name is instead Thai, Makrut, Wild, or Asian Lime. Find the double leaves at most markets, or if not available, look for them at an Asian market. Though the flavor will be slightly different, you can substitute Asian Lime leaves in a recipe with grated lime zest, dash of lime juice, and a bay leaf.

LOTUS ROOT

A root vegetable found underwater and similar in shape to a long squash. The skin is reddish brown in color; the inside is white and full of symmetrical holes that make slices look like snowflakes. You'll probably need to look for lotus root at an Asian grocery. I only use it for one recipe and recommend it as a pretty garnish, but it is optional.

DURIAN

The king of fruits, and my favorite ever. This fruit is found at Asian markets fresh, when in season, and is usually available frozen. If you can find it whole, it's about the size of a football and has wooden spikes on the exterior. You can also find frozen durian flesh packaged with seeds and bark removed. I use durian only for the Coconut Durian Shake recipe, and you can substitute any other fruit instead. To find out more about durian, watch the video I made in Bali: http://www.youtube.com/aniphyo#p/u/15/teV_F2GdwXI.

JACKFRUIT

Look for this at an Asian market, fresh when in season, or frozen. It tastes like bubble gum and is sticky. I use it in a jackfruit curry recipe, but you can substitute with your favorite vegetables instead.

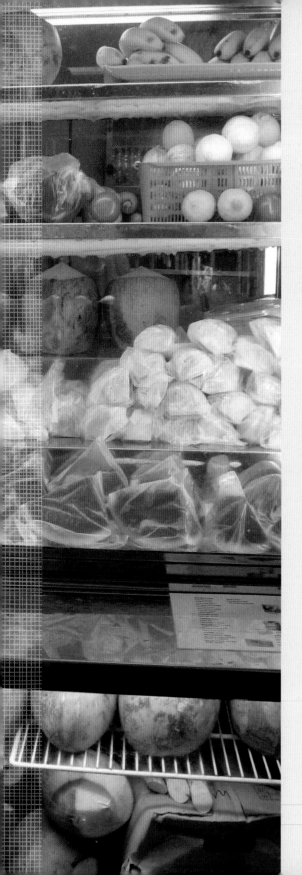

LYCHEE

Round, covered in a leathery reddish skin, and slightly smaller than an apricot. Lychee is sometimes available at natural food stores but is easier to find at an Asian market. I use it to fill a dessert crepe recipe, but it can be substituted with your favorite fruit.

SEEDS

I usually buy these in bulk. Look for raw labels and choose organic when possible. Available online at www.GoSuperLife.com.

SESAME SEEDS

Tan seeds and black seeds, if you can find it, but not necessary. Both tan and black are available at www.GoSuperLife.com.

FLAXSEEDS

Tan and/or brown.

BUCKWHEAT GROATS

When buckwheat seeds, which have a unique triangular shape, are dehulled (the outer hull removed), the remaining seed material is the groat. Buckwheat is not a cereal grain nor a wheat and is free of wheat gluten. It's energizing and nutritious and lower in fat than nuts and high in protein. I soak groats overnight, rinse well, then dry completely in a dehydrator for three to five hours at 104°F and store in a glass jar. These Buckwheat Crispies (page 247) can be sprinkled over salads, soups, in wraps, ground into a flour, and used to make a breakfast porridge. Look for groats labeled raw and hulled.

OAT GROATS

Raw and hulled. Oats are a seed, have a high fiber content, are high in potassium, protein, calcium, and B vitamins. The soluble fiber helps lower cholesterol by slowing absorption of glucose in the body. Only one recipe in the desserts section of this book calls for oat groats, and they can also be soaked overnight and processed with banana or dates to make a delicious morning porridge.

NUTS

Look for raw nuts, and as always, organic when possible. Available online at www.GoSuper Life.com.

- Cashews
- Almonds
- Pine nuts
- Pistachio
- Walnuts
- Coconut, dried shredded

BUTTERS

All nut and seed butters should be labeled raw; also choose organic when possible. There are many different butters available, but I use only two in this book. Available online at: www .GoSuperLife.com.

- Tahini
- Almond butter

SPICES AND SEASONINGS

I buy these in bulk, and organic whenever possible.

- Cardamom, ground
- Coriander, ground
- Cumin, ground
- Turmeric, ground
- Curry powder
- Cayenne powder

- Chile flakes
- Saffron threads
- Vanilla extract or vanilla beans (alcohol-free vanilla extract, or whole beans)
- Apple cider vinegar (Raw, look for filaments at the bottom of the bottle as a sign of live enzymes. Available at all grocery stores and at www.GoSuperLife.com.)
- Sea salt (fine and coarse, available at all grocery stores and at www.GoSuperLife.com)

VEGAN REFRIGERATED INGREDIENTS
Usually found in the same area as vegan fake meats and soy cheeses.

MISO PASTE
Look for miso labeled unpasteurized, non-GMO, and preferably organic. White or red, but any color will work.

KELP NOODLES
Made from the sea vegetable kelp. They're clear, have about 6 calories per serving, are low-carb with about 1 gram per serving, and have a mild flavor that works great in all noodle recipes. Can be substituted with spiralized vegetable noodles or coconut meat cut into noodle strips.

OILS
Whenever possible, choose organic.

TOASTED SESAME SEED OIL
Has a distinct Asian flavor but is not raw. Can be substituted with raw sesame oil.

COCONUT OIL
Look for virgin coconut oil (VCO); avoid refined, bleached, and deodorized (RBD). VCO has the flavors and scent of fresh coconut. RBD is tasteless with no odor. Available at grocery and natural food stores, and at www.GoSuperLife.com.

OLIVE OIL
Extra-virgin cold pressed.

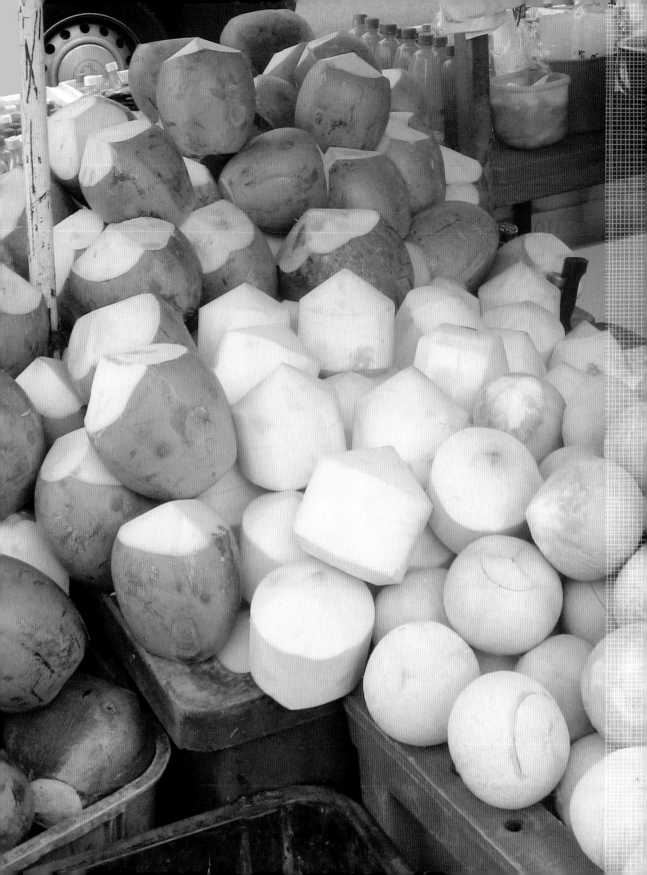

SWEETENERS

Choose whichever syrup(s) work for you, if any. As I've said in *Ani's Raw Food Kitchen*, I don't believe any bottled syrup is raw. They're all processed into a clear syrup. It's always best to go straight to Mother Nature by sweetening with whole fruits like dates, raisins, banana, or orange. I'll show you how to make your own Date Syrup on page 43. For blended recipes, you can substitute about one date to 1 tablespoon syrup, and then adjust to taste.

I use syrups in moderation for convenience, flavor, and consistency. I prefer agave or brown rice syrup for its mild color and flavor. Yacon is rich in color and flavor and great to use in the same way as molasses. Try using maple syrup, which has a distinct flavor, and always choose organic when possible.

I love stevia. The leaves of the stevia plant are dried and ground into a powder. Stevia has a distinct flavor you'll either like or not. Stevia has zero calories and doesn't register in the body as sugar at all. So give it a try and decide for yourself.

Most of these sweeteners are available online at www.GoSuperLife.com.

- Dates
- Agave syrup
- Yacon syrup
- Maple syrup (Choose Grade B, which is less refined than A)
- Rice syrup (Popular in macrobiotic diets, it's made with brown rice and an enzyme to transform the steamed grain into a sweet syrup.)
- Stevia (Look for powder, ideally green dried and ground leaves. White works, too, but is more processed. I love stevia because it's noncaloric and doesn't register in the body as a sugar.)
- Honey, raw (A vegan friend of mine will argue honey is vegan, especially since he is a beekeeper and rescues bees from extermination, brings them to his land, and gives them another hive. Others say it's not vegan because it is produced by bees, for bees. Whichever way you lean in this debate, raw honey's the most natural form of sweetener, has rich flavor, is antibacterial, antiviral, antifungal, contains antioxidants, and boosts our immune system.)

SHOPPING CHECKLIST

ASIAN AISLE

Arame

Dulse

Wakame

Nori

Korean chile powder and flakes, or cayenne
    powder and chile flakes

Nama Shoyu

Bragg Liquid Aminos

Tamari

Goji berries—12 to 16 ounces

Dried shiitake mushrooms

PRODUCE

*Buy fresh produce as needed per recipe on your
menu. I do like to keep a couple of coconuts on
hand at all times in the fridge.*

Thai young coconut—two or more

SEEDS

Sesame seeds—tan and black, if available

Flax—tan and/or brown

Buckwheat groats

NUTS

Cashews

Almonds

Pine nuts

Pistachio

Walnuts

Coconut, dried shredded

BUTTERS

Tahini

Almond butter

SPICES AND SEASONINGS

Start with about 2 ounces of each ground spice.

Cardamom, ground

Coriander, ground

Cumin, ground

Turmeric, ground

Curry powder

Cayenne powder

Chile flakes

Saffron threads

Vanilla extract, alcohol-free, or vanilla beans

Apple cider vinegar

Sea salt

VEGAN REFRIGERATED ITEMS

Miso paste

Kelp noodles—two 12-ounce bags, or more

OILS

Toasted sesame seed oil

Coconut oil (VCO)—virgin coconut oil

Extra-virgin olive oil

SWEETENERS

Dates, Medjool

Agave syrup

Yacon syrup

Maple syrup—Grade B

Brown rice syrup

Stevia—green or white powder

Honey, raw

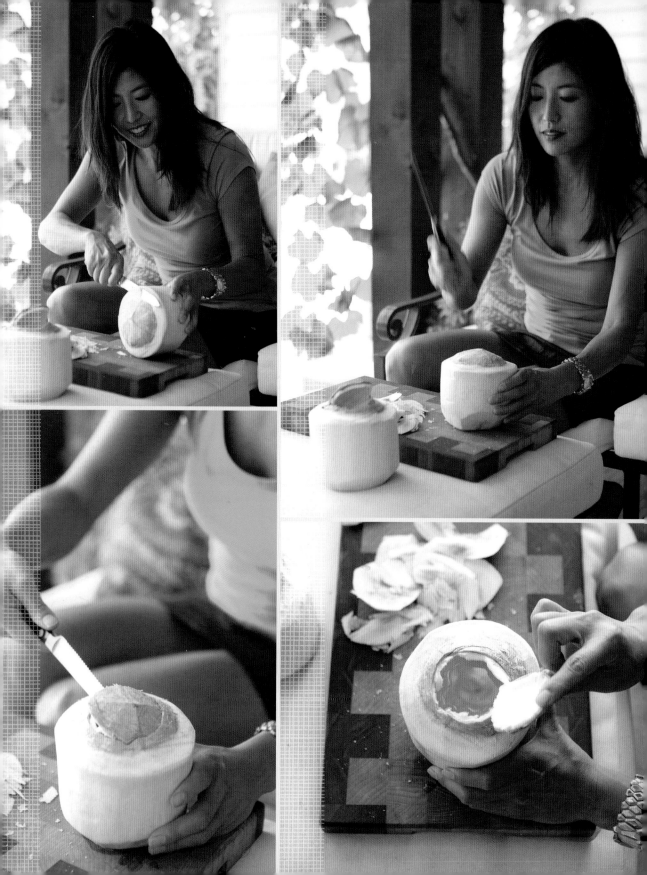

Techniques

OPENING A COCONUT

I've found an easy way to open up a coconut, which I teach in *Ani's Raw Food Essentials*, page 55.

1. Lay the coconut on its side. Use a knife to shave the white pith off the pointed top end until hard center is fully exposed (it looks like smooth wood).
2. Set the coconut upright. Use the heel of knife to gently tap around the edge of hard exposed center. The coconut has a natural stress line around the crown that will give and crack open.
3. Place the heel of the knife in the opening and rock back and forth to split open a circular opening.
4. Pull back and remove the top from the coconut. Pour coconut water into a container. Drink immediately or set aside and refrigerate for use later.

Now that the coconut is open and the water has been removed, scrape out coconut meat with a strong, large spoon. Hold the spoon's curve opposite the coconut's curve, upside down compared to how we hold when eating soup. I like to see if I can get all the meat out in one piece. Place meat in a bowl and clean by running your fingers over it to remove any hard pieces.

SPIRALIZING NOODLES

It's easy to make angel hair–shaped noodles using vegetables like zucchini, beets, carrots, and daikon radish. The machine is a bit finicky, so be patient at first, and before you know it you'll have beautiful vegetable noodles to enjoy! (See photos on next page.)

1. Cut the vegetable in 3½-inch lengths with flat ends.
2. Turn blade to the setting for thin noodles.
3. Place vegetable onto the small pin in your spiral slicer and secure top.
4. Press firmly while rotating handle slowly to make spiral noodles.

SLICING, CUTTING, CRUSHING

I like to use a chef's knife that's about 6 to 8 inches long to slice, julienne, cube, dice, and mince.

SLICE

Always curl your fingertips under, away from blade. Press straight down slicing into the food to get pieces the thickness you want. A mandoline slicer will slice paper-thin slices. Your food processor with slicing attachment will slice super fast.

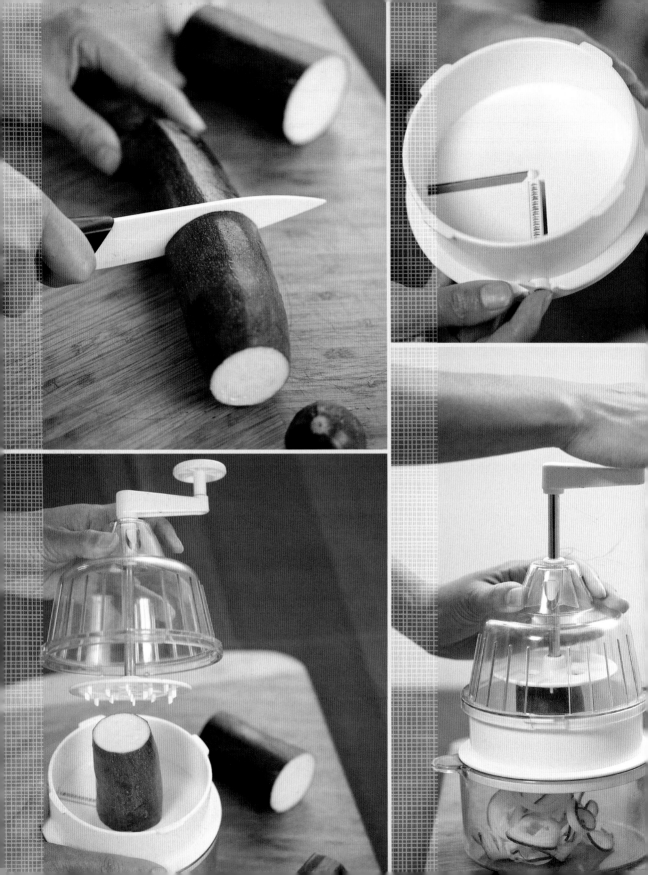

JULIENNE (MATCHSTICK)

Technically, matchsticks measure ⅛ inch by ⅛ inch by 1 to 2 inches. A fun tool to look for is a julienne slicer. It looks like a vegetable peeler, but with teeth, allowing you to "peel" thin, long strips. To julienne with a knife, follow these easy steps:

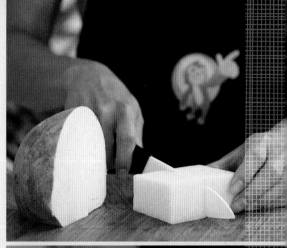

1. Cut into 1- to 2-inch segments, then square off edges so you're left with a rectangle.
2. Cut thin, even slices, and stack them.
3. Slice down through stack to create bundle of thin matchstick strips.

CUBE, DICE, OR MINCE

Cube, dice, and mince differ by the size of the squares cut. Cube has the largest squares, dice is between ⅛ to ¼ inch in size, and mince is about 1/16 of an inch.

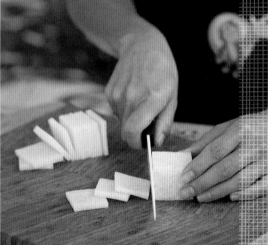

Chopping allows ingredients to retain their character and flavor, while diced ingredients, being smaller, will have a milder impact. Since herbs are strongly flavored, you don't want them to be concentrated in large chunks. Mincing into small squares helps them blend into the overall dish.

To cube, dice, or mince with your knife, follow these easy steps:

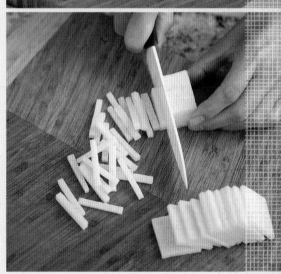

1. Cut into long sticks by using julienne technique
2. Cut across sticks to create cubes you want

CRUSH

Crushing ginger or garlic releases essential oils and flavor.

1. To crush garlic, place a clove onto a cutting board. Lay knife over garlic horizontally, making sure the sharp blade edge faces away from you.
2. Press flat part of blade down firmly with free hand to crush garlic underneath. Remove skin. (You may choose to mince your crushed clove before using.)

SHRED, GRATE, ZEST

Shredding makes the largest pieces, grating makes a chunky powder texture, and zesting is like grating citrus skin.

SHRED

To shred is to slice into small pieces, like shredding carrots for a carrot cake or cabbage for coleslaw. Place vegetable against surface of shredder, like the box style used for dairy cheese, and rub back and forth to shred. The food processor and mandoline slicer have attachments for shredding, and the food processor makes shredding really fast.

GRATE

Using a micro planer makes grating and zesting easy. Just rub ginger back and forth along surface of your grater and catch shavings in a bowl or on a flat surface.

ZEST

Rub unpeeled citrus fruit across micro planer or zester to grate off only the exterior of the peel. Avoid the white pith, which tastes bitter.

SOAKING AND SPROUTING

SOAKING

The easiest way I soak is to simply place nuts and seeds into at least double the amount of filtered water overnight. In the morning, I rinse the nuts and seeds well and discard the soaking water. If you really want to get into it, there are specific soaking times for different seeds and nuts, but I like taking the easiest route possible.

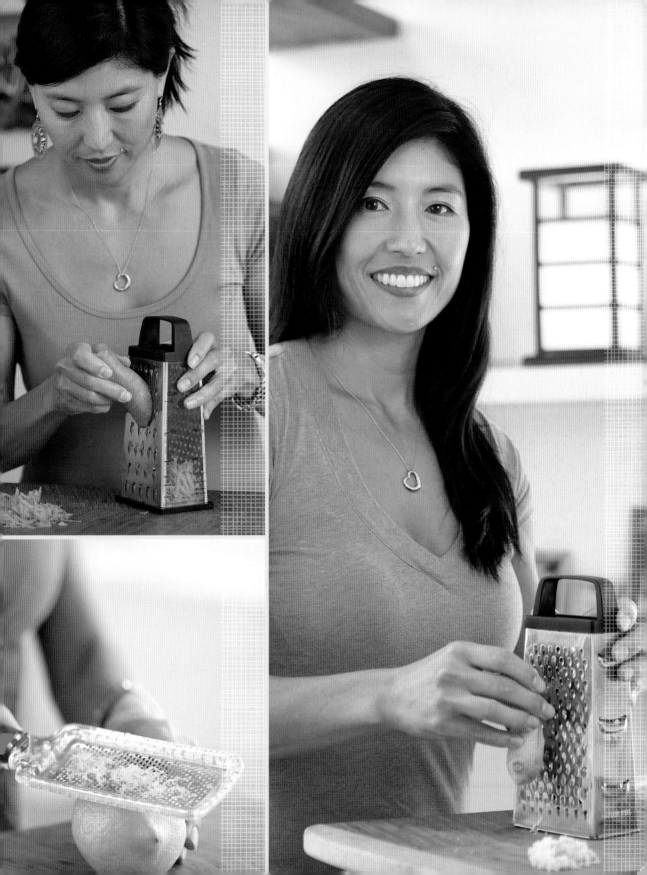

I find it easiest to drain soaked nuts and seeds through a fine-mesh sieve after rinsing. To sprout them, I'll keep them in the sieve, balanced over a bowl or container, until I see a small tail starting to sprout. Depending on the nut or seed, this can take from hours to days. I run water over the sieve to rinse the nuts or seeds a few times throughout the day.

The benefits of soaking and sprouting are that they begin the germination process in the dormant nut or seed, making it easier to digest and converting the carbohydrates to protein. When I'm traveling and on the road, it's impossible for me to soak or sprout, so I'll forego it then, and do the best I can when I'm at home.

Ideally, you want to soak all nuts and seeds before using them in your recipes. But again, do the best you can. I find that lately I have less time for soaking and sprouting than I used to.

SPROUTING

Growing sprouts is an easy way to have an indoor garden all year round. The Chinese were known to carry mung beans on sea journeys away from land. They sprouted and ate sprouts to avoid scurvy from vitamin C deficiency. Sprouts are high in vitamins A, B, C, D, E, and K. They're a good source of all amino acids, calcium, chlorophyll, zinc, iron, magnesium, and contain up to 35 percent protein.

You can find sprouting seeds at your local natural food store and online. Different types of sprouting seeds are available at www.GoSuperLife.com.

DAY 1

1. To grow most small seeds into sprouts, place 2 tablespoons of seeds into a 1-quart wide-mouth jar. Cover with mesh nylon tulle from a fabric store or cheesecloth, and secure with a rubber band. Add filtered water to rinse, swirl, and drain.
2. Soak seeds by adding 2 cups of filtered water to the jar and soak seeds for eight to twelve hours at room temperature. Soaking before bed makes it simple. Keep jars away from sunlight.

DAY 2

3. Rinse seeds two times a day, morning and evening, by refilling the jar with filtered water, swirling, and draining. Turn the jar upside down and prop at a 45-degree angle on a dish rack to allow air flow and draining.

DAYS 3 TO 6

4. Continue to rinse seeds and sprouts two times a day, tip and set at 45 degrees to drain and breathe. In three to six days, you'll see sprouts beginning to grow.

5. When green leaves begin to grow on the sprouts, move jar to a brighter location, but not into direct sunlight.

6. Your sprouts are ready to eat when they are 1 to 2 inches long, about double the length of the seeds.

I take the easy route and soak the nuts and seeds overnight. If you want to follow more specific instructions, here's a general chart to work from:

SEED OR NUT DRY AMOUNT	SOAKING TIME	SPROUTING TIME	SPROUTED YIELD
Almonds, 1 cup	8–10 hours	1–2 days, if sproutable	2 cups
Pecans, Walnuts, 1 cup	4–6 hours	1–2 days	2 cups
Cashews, 1 cup	4–6 hours	1–2 days, if sproutable	2 cups
Buckwheat, 1 cup	6 hours	2 days	2 cups
Pumpkin seeds, 1 cup	6–8 hours	1 day	2 cups
Sesame seeds (hulled only), 1 cup	4–6 hours	1–2 days	1 cup
Sunflower seeds, 1 cup	6–10 hours	1 day	2 cups
Flax seeds, 1 cup	4–6 hours	1 day	2 cups
Oat groats, 1 cup	6 hours	2 days	2 cups
Quinoa, 1 cup	2–3 hours	1 day	3 cups

To store, cover jar, or transfer sprouts to a container and cover. Refrigerate and enjoy for up to a week.

Always rinse sprouts before use and discard slimy sprouts or any that smell off. When sprouts have grown to the size you like, store in refrigeration to slow further growth and to prevent decay and mold. Keep sprouts rinsed and drained, and use within a week.

Food safety agencies have issued warnings about sprouts harboring various harmful bacteria, especially when handled commercially by numerous people. Food safety is all the more reason for growing your own sprouts, as well as shopping locally and seasonally as much as possible.

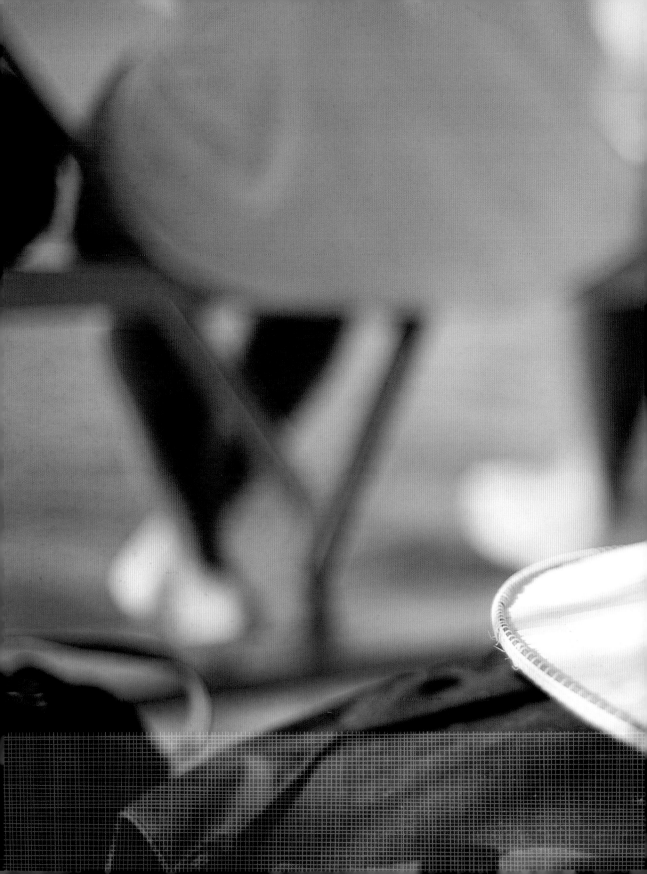

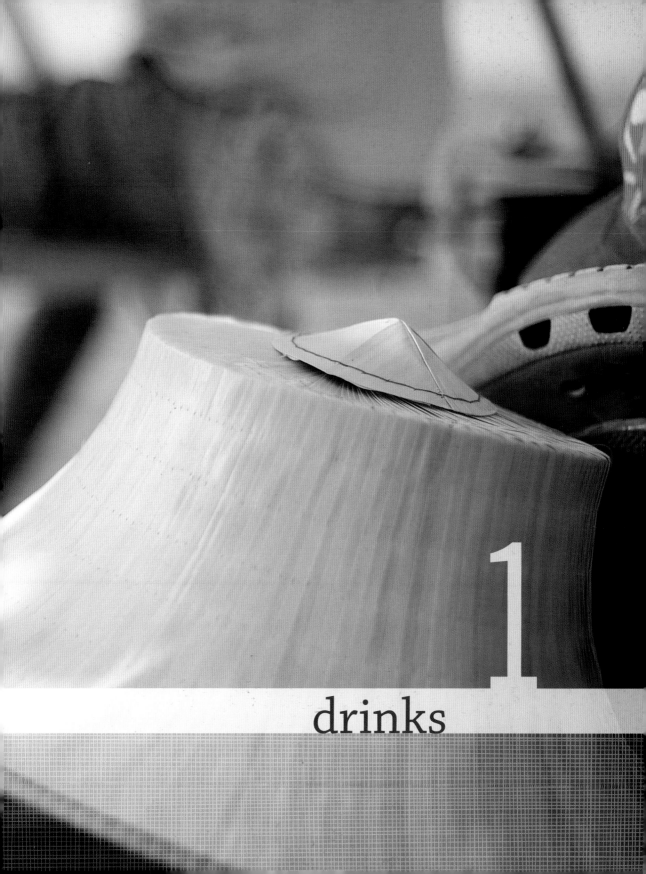

1

drinks

Entertaining in the Raw

I cherish the time I get to spend with good friends and family, sharing stories, laughing, singing, dancing, and creating lasting memories together. I love serving up raw foods when entertaining because my friends and family think it's delicious, and because I know it's super healthy and will help them live long lives. I'm on my path toward longevity, and I want to ensure my friends and family will hang around for a long time with me.

Raw foods are the perfect food for entertaining in a snap. When a friend calls to say she just arrived in town and will be over in thirty minutes, that may not be enough time to cook something, but that's more than enough time to whip up a platter of beautiful raw snacks. It's as easy as blending, processing, plating, and serving.

Quick and fresh, these recipes offer an easy way to use everyday, easy-to-find vegetables with Asian spices and herbs like basil, mint, cilantro, cardamom, and spicy chile to create tantalizing flavors and hours of engaging conversation.

Even for the morning after, when we do partake of a bit too much to drink, Asian foods are great for curing hangovers. The chile, fresh herbs, and spices are naturally detoxifying and cleansing and help us clean up and recover from the night before.

SAMPLE MENUS

In chapter 10 of this book, I include sample menus for throwing a brunch with family and friends, inviting people over for a cocktail or dinner party, planning a picnic for a Sunday afternoon, celebrating a wedding, and hosting a potluck or buffet. In addition, I give some menu-planning ideas for birthdays and other celebrations and for dreaming up a romantic dinner for a date. I even list a few recipes that make thoughtful post-party take-home gifts.

WINE PAIRING

The full, fresh flavors in my Asian raw recipes make wine pairing easy. Recipes with shiitake mushrooms, for example, go well with an earthy Pinot Noir, while lemon and citrus go well with a Sauvignon Blanc. Consider pairing opposites like a hot or spicy curry with a sweet dessert wine. Opposing flavors can work off each other to create new flavor experiences while cleansing the palate.

In the same way I prefer choosing local and seasonal produce, I like to match my geographic location to the wine. Regional foods and wines that have developed together over time have a natural affinity for each other. I also choose wine that's organic and biodynamic. Biodynamic is a supercharged system of organic farming. Not only are synthetic fertilizers and pesticides avoided, soil is considered a living organism, and its overall health is taken into consideration. The cycles and balance of

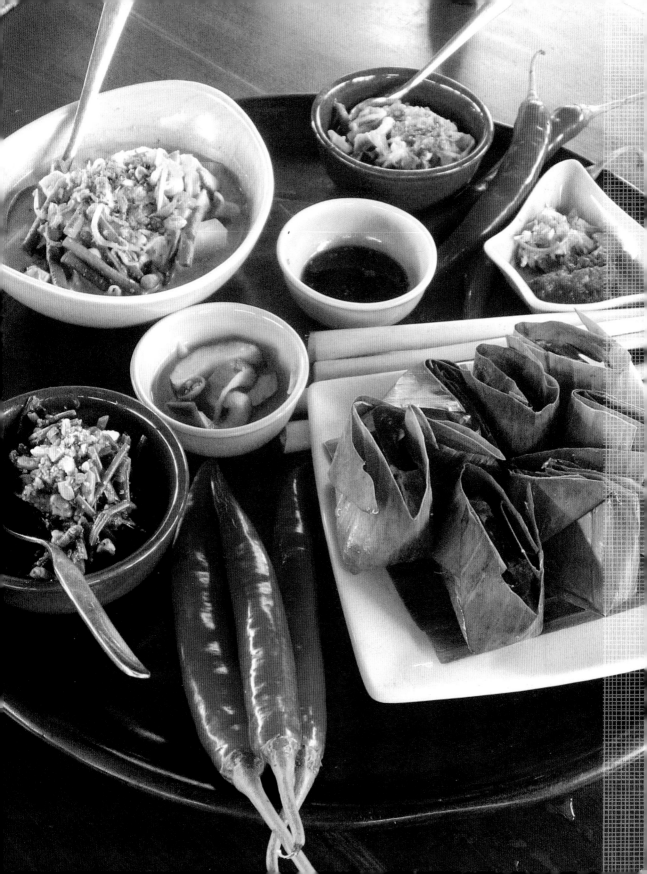

ORGANIC VS. BIODYNAMIC

Wine labeled as "100% organic" is made using 100 percent organically grown ingredients and contains only naturally occurring sulfites in less than 100 parts per million. Wine labeled "organic" means it is made of at least 95 percent organic ingredients, that the remaining portion of the ingredients are elements that are not available organically, and that its naturally occurring sulfites are less than 100ppm. A wine label that says the wine is "made with organic grapes" will not carry the USDA organic logo and will be made with at least 70 percent organic ingredients plus added artificial sulfites to a maximum of 100ppm. Finally, wine labeled "biodynamic" is not only 100 percent organic but is created in an environment that is aligned with the processes and cycles of nature. The biodynamic vineyard is seen as a complete living system with insects, plants, and animals that live and work together in the vineyard to create amazing tasting wines.

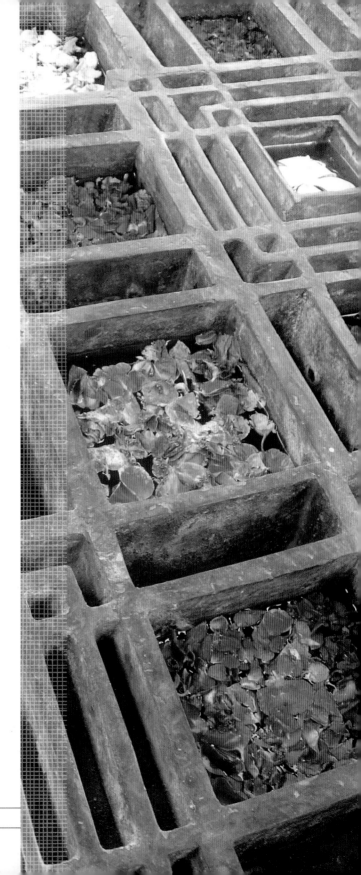

nature are considered, as well as how the stars and planets affect the timing for farming processes. Biodynamic wine growers usually make their own compost.

Sweetness in a dish accentuates the bitterness and astringency in wine to make it taste drier, stronger, and less fruity. Try pairing a Riesling with cardamom, lavender, coconut, or citrus and a Moscato D'Asti or a late-harvest Viognier from California with fresh or dried fruit.

Acidity in a dish from citrus or vinegar will lessen the sourness of a wine, making it taste richer, mellower, and sweeter. Choose an acidic wine when pairing with a milder dish like a white Sauvignon Blanc or a sparkling wine. Or, a Chianti for fuller-flavored dishes.

Bitter flavors from bitter greens like chicory and citrus peel accentuate the bitter, tannic elements in wine. Pair with a bitter red wine like a Cabernet Sauvignon, Merlot, Zinfandel, or Syrah.

Salt in food will tone down the bitterness and astringency in wine, making sweet wines taste sweeter. Acidity in wine cuts saltiness in food making a sparkling wine good for pairing.

Enjoy wine, if partaking, in balance. Celebrations and gatherings are about laughter and creating memories to add into our memory banks. Excessive alcohol harms our body's immune system. Like sugar, alcohol in excess reduces the ability of white cells to multiply to kill germs and cancer. One drink doesn't seem to dampen our immune system, but three or more drinks do.

ECO ENTERTAINING

I love dancing, but my favorite styles of music don't start playing until well after midnight, and usually on a weekday. Even though raw food gives me lots of energy, I'm usually in bed before the DJ starts spinning. I prefer throwing parties earlier in the day and encourage my friends to do the same for selfish reasons, so I can attend! My favorite is a Sunday afternoon party in the park because it is solar powered, and I get to soak up the sun, too.

You can eco entertain in style by catering with my organic, raw recipes. The biggest impact we have on our planet is through our food choices. Eating vegan, organic, and raw leaves the lightest footprint on our planet. Choose organic and biodynamic wines. Get an accurate head count so you make the right amount of food without waste. And, let guests take home leftovers you won't be able to eat quickly enough.

Choose a centrally located venue that's easy to get to by public transportation and suggest and help coordinate carpooling. Shuttle guests in a large car or charter a bus to a venue that's far away.

On beautiful summer nights, consider putting food outdoors to take advantage of the natural light. When choosing candles, buy beeswax, soy, or vegetable. Reusable tableware is always preferred, and renting or borrowing flatware and stemware is something to consider. For disposable options, look for plates and utensils made from fast-growing bamboo (manufacturers say bamboo will decompose in six months), plates made from sugarcane fiber, PLA plastic made from corn (industrially

CHINESE SYMBOLISM

Asians love big, beautiful, and fresh fruits. Fresh fruit at the New Year symbolizes life and a new beginning. Sugared fruits are used as a wish for a sweet year ahead. Fruits are common gifts and common temple offerings.

The orange is a prayer or wish for good fortune and is the most common food offering. Two mandarins are given to a new bride to share with her husband on their wedding night to symbolize the family's wish for the bride and groom to share a happy and full life together. Mandarin in Cantonese means "gold," adding wishes for a prosperous life together.

Large melons and pomelo are shared by the members of a family and are symbolic of family unity to stay round, large, whole, and united. Pomegranates are full of seeds inside and symbolize fertility. Bananas on a table or altar symbolize a wish for education and brilliance at work and school. Apples symbolize peace.

Peaches represent long life. The wood of the peach tree is said to ward off evil, while the petals of the blossoms were known to put men into an intense trance of love.

Bamboo is a Chinese symbol for longevity because it's durable, strong, flexible, and resilient, surviving the harshest conditions and standing tall and green year round. The flexibility and adaptability of bamboo teach us that the secret to a long happy life is to go with the flow.

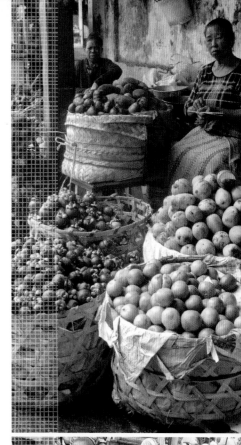

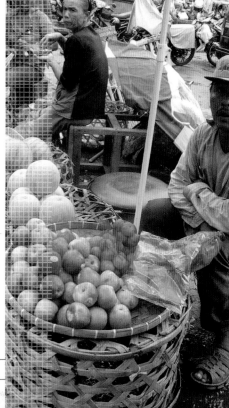

compostable), or PET plastic with the recycling code 1, because it is the easiest plastic to recycle. I like to avoid washing a gazillion dishes and opt for using the same plate for most, if not all, the meal. Flatware can be licked clean between courses.

After the party's over, clean up and save anything you can reuse. Package leftovers to take into the office to share with coworkers the next day. Use your dishwasher if it's fully loaded and your detergent is earth-friendly, nontoxic, and phosphate-free. A fully loaded dishwasher is said to be more efficient than washing all those dishes by hand. Turn off the dry cycle and air dry instead.

Nut Mylks

It's very easy to make your own fresh nut mylk. Just place a handful of your favorite nut (ideally soaked overnight and rinsed well) into a high speed blender, then add coconut or filtered water, and blend smooth. This makes for a fresh mylk alternative to traditional dairy milk and making your own is economical, too.

Many other cultures don't rely on dairy milk as we do in America; homemade nut mylks provide protein and rich flavor—without the excess packaging or processing.

THE SOY STORY

In Korea, you won't find milk, or dairy for that matter. Instead, we have soy milk and tofu as our cheese, which are both used as condiments in small quantities, rather than as main dishes. In America, soy is the number-one pesticide-laden crop. It's also commonly genetically modified, unless it says non-GMO. So, chances are, if you are eating soy in America, you're eating a lot of poison—yet another reason to make your own fresh nut mylks.

Mother Jones published an article on soy burgers in America containing hexane, an EPA-registered air pollutant and neurotoxin poison. You can read it about it here: http://motherjones.com/blue-marble/2010/04/veggie-burgers-neurotoxin-hexane

DATE SYRUP

People now realize agave syrup is fructose and, therefore, basically the same and maybe worse for our health than high-fructose corn syrup, though both are technically low glycemic. I have always promoted avoiding or using in moderation all things processed. As is true of all bottled syrups, agave syrup is manufactured and processed. The healthiest way to sweeten is to use a date syrup that you make yourself (see next page).

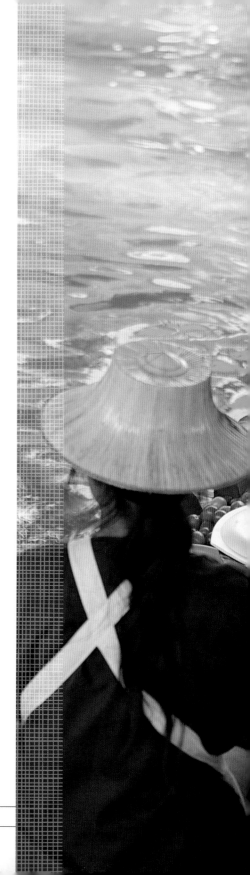

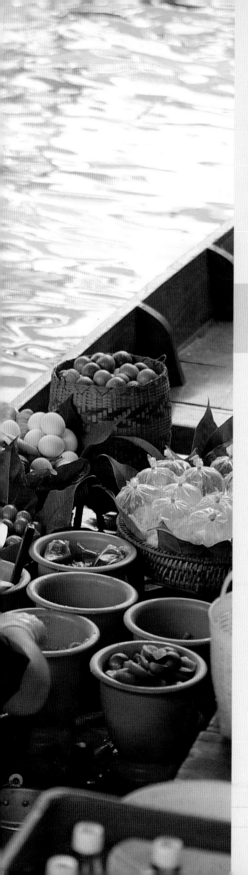

DATE SYRUP
India

MAKES 1 CUP

It's simple to make Date Syrup. All you need are your favorite dates and a blender. I choose soft or semi-soft dates, like Khadrawy or Medjool. If using a drier date, use the water in the recipe to soak the dates first until soft, about 30 minutes or longer.

½ cup pitted dates
½ to 1 cup filtered water, as desired

Place pitted dates and water in blender, blend smooth. Add as much water as you like for desired consistency.

VARIATIONS: *For different flavors of Date Syrup try the following:*

- *Use an orange (whole, seeded, and peeled) instead of the water, and add additional water only as needed.*

- *Substitute filtered water for Rose Water (page 255).*

- *Add 1 tablespoon cacao or carob powder, the seeds of a vanilla bean, or 1 tablespoon vanilla extract.*

- *Add lavender or mint extracts, to taste.*

NUT AND SEED MYLK
India

MAKES 4 SERVINGS

Cashews are a sweeter nut by nature, and when I make cashew mylk, I often leave out any sweetener. But if you like your mylk on the sweeter side, sweeten with stevia, agave syrup, or a whole fruit like dates. Sesame seeds make for a calcium-packed mylk but can taste a bit bitter, so you may want to mix in some cashew or almond with it. Have fun exploring different nuts and mixes to make endless varieties of mylk.

½ cup of your favorite nuts and/or seeds, soaked in filtered water (see soaking table, page 33) and rinsed well before using

Pinch of stevia, or ⅓ cup pitted dates, or 3 tablespoons agave syrup, brown rice, or maple syrup, optional

Pinch of sea salt

5 cups coconut and/or filtered water

Place all ingredients into your blender, adding a small amount of water first. Blend smooth. Then, add remaining water and blend. I love fiber in my mylk, but you can always strain it out using a nut mylk or filtering bag if preferred.

Will keep for 4 days or longer in fridge.

VARIATIONS: *Add cacao powder, vanilla bean, or strawberries to make different flavored mylks. The possibilities truly are endless.*

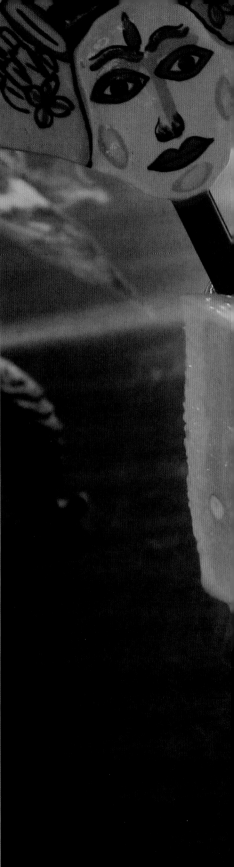

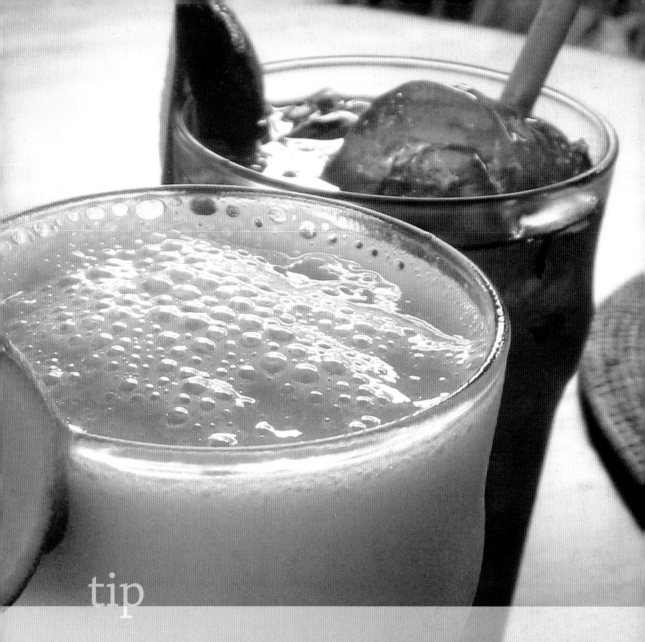

tip

 On cold mornings when I crave a hot chocolate mylk, I'll heat up my drink in a saucepan while using my finger to check when it's warmed up to my liking. That's usually when it feels warm to my touch, which is about 104 degrees.

Tea

Tea can be steeped in the sun in a glass jar to make sun tea. Just place your favorite bags of tea in filtered water, and place your jar in the sun for a few hours, until brewed to your liking. The Korean-inspired tea below steeps a dried fig instead of tea leaves.

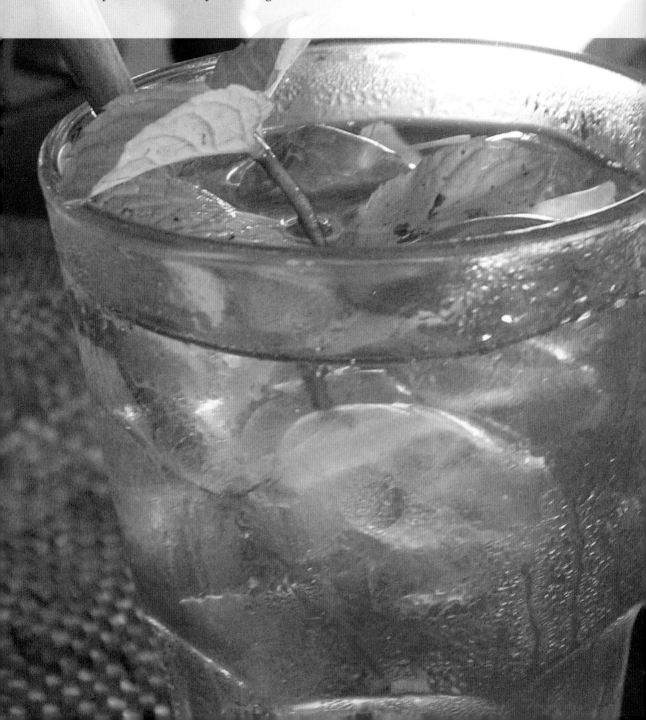

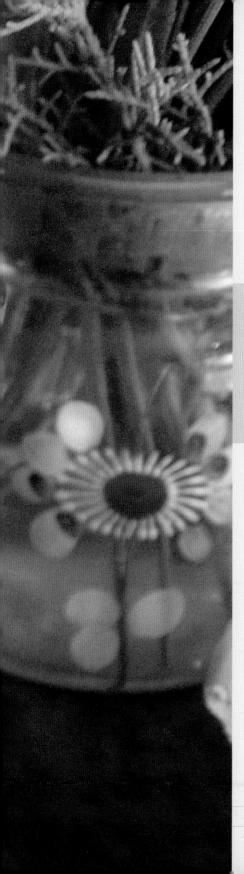

CINNAMON, FIG, AND GINGER SUN TEA

Korea

MAKES 4 SERVINGS

This is a sweet and spicy tea thought to help fight colds and reduce stress. It's typically made with dried persimmons, which can be hard to find, so I use Calimyrna figs instead. You can substitute with your favorite dried fig. Traditionally served chilled, but can also be enjoyed warm.

3 cups filtered water

4 teaspoons fresh julienned ginger

¼ teaspoon ground cinnamon

2 tablespoons agave or brown rice syrup, or pinch of stevia

4 dried Calimyrna figs

1 tablespoon pine nuts, for garnish

Place all ingredients, except the pine nuts, into a large glass jar. Set in the sun for a few hours to "brew" and for the figs to hydrate.

Serve chilled or warmed. Pour into four cups, placing one of the soaked figs into each. Top with pine nuts and serve immediately.

Shakes

Shakes are made by blending together fruit like avocado, mango, or durian with water, coconut milk, or coconut water. Coconut is actually a fruit, though the FDA defines it as a nut for labeling purposes. All of the shakes below are free of nuts.

Coconut is a great source of electrolytes, and coconut water makes for a great post-workout drink.

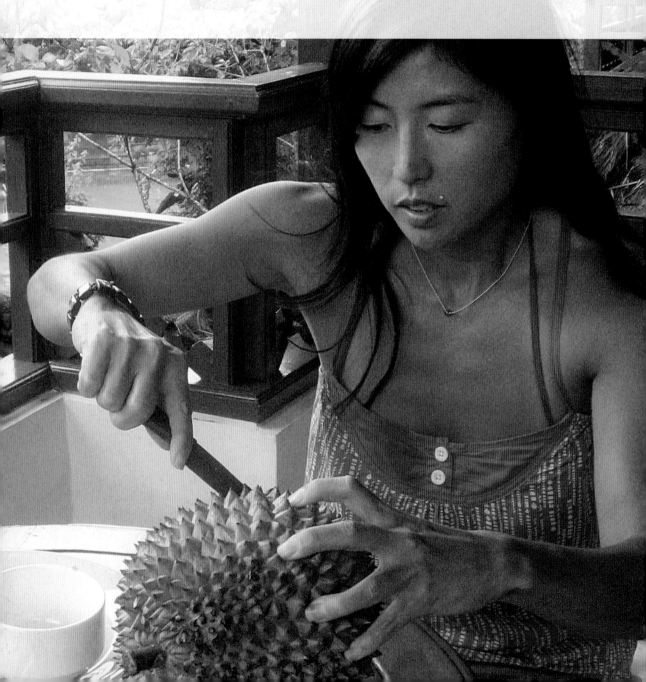

COCONUT DURIAN SHAKE
Thailand

MAKES 4 SERVINGS

I know durian is hardly a common, everyday ingredient here in the States. But, since durian is one of my favorite fruits, I had to include this recipe here. If you can't find durian, you can just use 3 cups of your favorite fruit in this recipe instead.

Durian is Mother Nature's custard, and is a fatty fruit like avocado that's packed with sulfur and MSM (methylsulfonylmethane). Great for our joints and softening scar tissue, MSM is a powerful antioxidant that increases blood flow. Coconut also has twice the potassium of a banana. The electrolytes and potassium in coconut plus the MSM in durian make this smoothie great post-workout fuel.

If you don't know what a durian is and want to see what it looks like, check out the video I shot about durian in Bali: http://www.youtube.com/watch?v=teV_F2GdwXI.

3 cups deseeded durian flesh, fresh or frozen

2 coconuts, water and meat

¼ teaspoon cinnamon

Additional filtered water, as needed

Place durian, coconut water, coconut meat, and cinnamon into your blender. Blend smooth. Add additional water as desired to create the consistency you prefer.

Enjoy immediately.

SWEET STEVIA

Stevia is a plant; when you pick off its leaf and put it in your mouth, it tastes sweet. This natural sweetness won't register in your body as sugar at all, doesn't trigger insulin responses as other sweeteners do, and has such negligible calories it's considered noncaloric.

Stevia leaves are dried and ground down into a green powder. This powder is also found in white, but it takes more processing to make a green powder white. Stevia drops are available, but that means even more processing to manufacture a concentrated liquid. I prefer the green powder whenever I can find it. I keep intending to grow my own plant, which would be the best option of all.

Stevia has a particular flavor, so if you like it, feel free to substitute agave or maple syrup and other sweeteners with stevia instead. Keep in mind that 1 tablespoon of agave syrup can be replaced by just a pinch of stevia powder or a drop of the liquid. This works fine for smoothies. But, some recipes, like desserts, may need the syrup for its stickiness to help bind ingredients together.

If you're trying to decrease body fat while increasing muscle mass, you may want to cut back on sweeteners, fruits, and fats. It doesn't have to be about losing weight, but about striving for a stronger, leaner body. Personally, I love sweets, so stevia is a great substitute that helps me decrease calories and sugar intake.

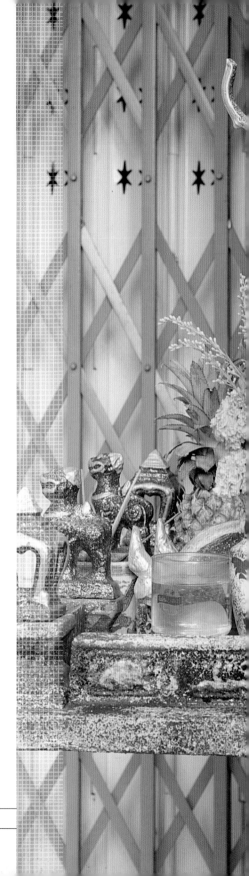

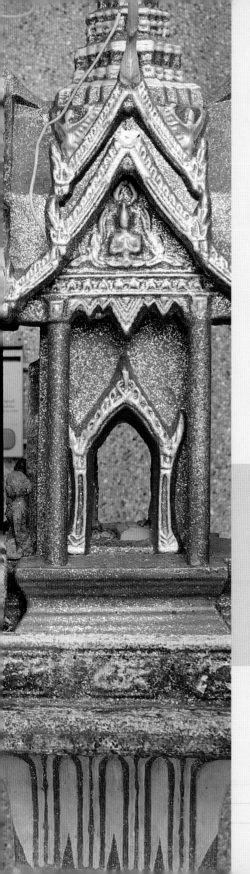

AVOCADO SHAKE WITH CHOCOLATE FUDGE SAUCE

Indonesia

MAKES 4 SERVINGS

I love all things green. So when I first saw this thick, creamy, green shake in Bali, I was drawn to it. Chocolate sauce drizzled down the inside of the glass adds both an aesthetic and flavor kick. In Bali, these shakes are often sweetened with sugar and so have that gritty, sugary crunch. I recommend adding your favorite sweetener, and enough of it. Using a palm sugar, which is dehydrated palm juice, or date sugar, will also give your shake that sugary grit without the guilt.

Dates are a whole fruit straight from Mother Nature. You can substitute the sweetener in this recipe with 3 or 4 tablespoons Date Syrup (page 43), but it will darken the color of your green shake.

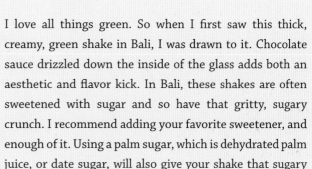

SHAKE

2 cups ripe avocado meat, from about 2 avocados

3 to 4 cups coconut milk (see page 144), as needed

1 cup ice

2 tablespoons agave syrup, or pinch of stevia, or 3 to 4 tablespoons Date Syrup (page 43), to taste

GARNISH

4 tablespoons Chocolate Fudge Sauce, optional (page 52)

Place all shake ingredients into your blender and blend smooth.

To serve, drizzle chocolate sauce around inside of glass first, if using. Then pour shake into your glass to create a pretty pattern. Enjoy immediately.

CHOCOLATE FUDGE SAUCE

Indonesia

MAKES ABOUT 1 CUP

This is the simple chocolate sauce from *Ani's Raw Food Essentials*, page 282. It's great as an accent to the avocado shake; it's also a delicious complement to ice kreams, desserts, or mixed into your favorite nut mylk for a sweet treat.

You can substitute Date Syrup in this recipe, but the texture of your syrup will be thicker from the fiber in the dates. It'll still taste delicious, though. For thinner consistency, add a splash of water, and to make it sweeter, add a pinch of stevia powder.

½ cup cacao powder

¾ cup agave, maple, or Date Syrup (page 43)

4 teaspoons extra-virgin olive oil

Blend all the ingredients together.

Will keep for a week or more in fridge.

MANGO LASSI

India

MAKES 4 SERVINGS

Fresh mango is blended with coconut milk, rose water, and cardamom. If you want to sweeten, use agave syrup or for fewer calories and less sugar, use a pinch of stevia. I like to add a few drops of rose water for a fragrant Indian touch.

If you don't have rose water on hand, use 2 cups Coconut Milk instead. If you have rose extract, add a drop or two.

3 cups peeled and diced ripe mango

1 cup Coconut Milk (page 144)

1 cup Rose Water (page 255)

1 tablespoon agave or Date Syrup (page 43), or a pinch of stevia powder, optional

¼ teaspoon ground cardamom

Place all ingredients in blender and blend smooth. Serve chilled or with ice.

Will keep for 1 day in the fridge.

SUPERFOOD COCONUT LEMONGRASS SMOOTHIE
Thailand

MAKES 4 SERVINGS

Antioxidant-laden superfoods like spirulina, matcha green tea, wheatgrass, maca, and lime give this smoothie its bright green color. Thai red chili gives it a spicy kick. The creamy texture comes from mango flavored with a hint of fresh lemongrass, blended with young Thai baby coconut meat. If you don't have coconut meat, you can add coconut flavor by using coconut oil instead, as noted in the recipe.

This smoothie is designed as a great pre- and post-workout fuel, or as a pick-me-up any time of the day. It's delicious and pumps you full of energy and nutrients to power you up. If you don't have every ingredient on hand, just using the mango, chile pepper, lemongrass, coconut meat or oil, and water will capture the key flavor and texture of this smoothie.

4 cups fresh or frozen mango, from 2 whole mangos, seeded and peeled

½ thai red chile pepper, to taste

4 inches of lemongrass, chopped

1 cup coconut meat from 1 to 2 Thai baby coconuts, or 2 tablespoons coconut oil

2 teaspoons spirulina powder

1 teaspoon matcha green tea powder

2 teaspoons wheatgrass powder, or 1½ tablespoons fresh

1 teaspoon maca powder

4 cups coconut water, or filtered water

Place all ingredients into your high-speed blender and blend smooth. Enjoy immediately.

FIVE FLAVORS OF LONGEVITY AND WELLNESS

Based on five basic flavors, Chinese Medicine uses food for healing: sour, sweet, bitter, spicy, and salty.

Sour acts as astringent for the intestines, will stop diarrhea, promotes salivation, quenches thirst, and moisturizes the body. Vinegar is used to prevent colds and cure cough.

Sweet tones the body, improves mood, and inhibits pain. Goji berries have been used for thousands of years to strengthen and build blood.

Bitter strengthens the stomach, promotes salivation, eliminates excess body heat, improves eyesight, and purges toxic substances. Almonds, celery, and kale are used to clear the lung and throat, lower blood pressure, and reduce inflammation.

Spicy foods can diffuse evil influence, moisten dryness, promote Qi (the circulating life energy inherent in all things) and blood circulation. Ginger, scallions, and garlic, and most spices are used to help sterilize food.

Salt softens firm masses and fibrous adhesions, purges and cleanses the colon, and is used for treating sores, inflammation, and cysts.

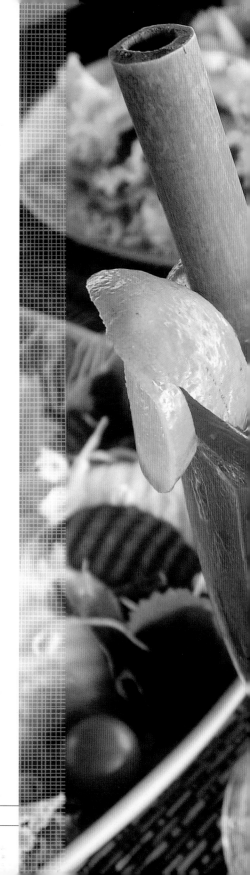

Cocktails

Cocktails are fun to serve when eco entertaining. They are bright in color, light, and full of flavor. The flavor profiles and colors of these cocktails are distinctly Asian, created with Asian ingredients and philosophy in mind. My cocktails are made with wine, but you can substitute with water kefir, coconut kefir, or sparkling water instead. Keep in mind moderation is key, especially when it comes to alcohol.

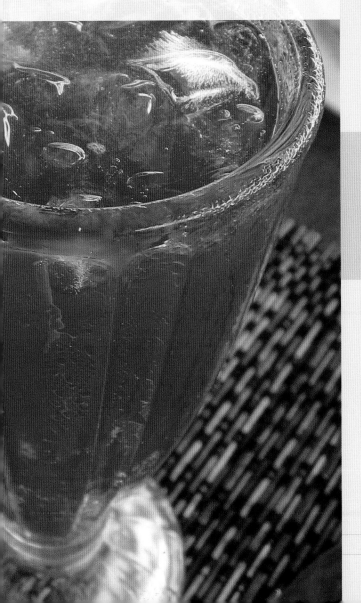

POMEGRANATE COCKTAIL

India

MAKES 4 SERVINGS

A bright red cocktail full of antioxidants from pomegranate with a hint of Asian lime leaf and sweet cardamom. Mix with white wine, or if you want to avoid alcohol, use sparkling water. I like to use my home brewed water kefir to support healthy digestion and elimination. You can find the recipe for brewing your own water kefir in *Ani's Raw Food Essentials*, page 54.

2 cups pomegranate juice

2 cups white wine, sparkling water, or water kefir

¼ teaspoon ground cardamom

¼ teaspoon very finely sliced Asian lime leaf

Into a martini shaker, place juice, wine, cardamom, and Asian lime leaves along with a few ice cubes and muddle to mix well.

Strain and pour into four martini glasses and enjoy immediately.

BLUSHING ROSES

Japan

MAKES 4 SERVINGS

A beautiful light pink drink with a hint of rose mixed with white wine or probiotic water kefir (check out the recipe in *Ani's Raw Food Essentials*, page 54). Serve with a wedge of lime.

2½ cups white wine or water kefir

1 cup rose water, or 1 cup filtered water with 1 or 2 drops of rose extract

½ cup pomegranate juice

Lime wedges, for garnish

In martini shaker, add white wine, rose water, and pomegranate juice and shake to chill.

Pour into four cocktail glasses and garnish with wedge of lime.

COSMOJITOS

Vietnam

MAKES 4 SERVINGS

Flavors and colors of lime, mint, pineapple, and orange fuse with white wine or water kefir to make a beautifully refreshing cocktail that's fun for celebrating life.

1 lime, peeled and seeded

1 tablespoon mint leaves

1 cup pineapple chunks

1 cup peeled and seeded orange (about 1 large orange)

3 cups white wine or water kefir

Place all ingredients into blender, blend smooth. Add about a cup of ice, and blend to chill.

Strain and pour into four cocktail glasses.

VANILLA JALAPEÑO COCKTAIL

Thailand

MAKES 4 SERVINGS

White wine or water kefir with a kiss of vanilla and the kick of spicy jalapeño. I love spice because it's warming and gets my blood pumping. Capsaicin in spicy peppers is known to help us burn fat and lose weight. Vanilla has the most amazing scent, making it an aphrodisiac that lifts our spirits.

4 cups white wine or water kefir

1 vanilla bean, scraped, or 1 tablespoon vanilla extract, alcohol-free

¼ teaspoon sliced jalapeño, to taste

4 slices jalapeño, for garnish

Place all ingredients into cocktail shaker and muddle to mix well.

Strain and pour into four cocktail glasses, garnish with a slice of jalapeño. Enjoy immediately.

FRESH LEMONADE COCKTAIL

Hawaii

MAKES 4 SERVINGS

A simple cocktail of white wine or water kefir mixed together with fresh lemon juice to make a cool, refreshing drink.

3 cups white wine or water kefir

¾ cup coconut or filtered water

¼ cup lemon juice, fresh

Pinch of stevia or 2 tablespoons of agave, maple, or brown rice syrup

Place all ingredients into cocktail shaker with a couple cubes of ice. Shake to mix and to chill.

Pour into four cocktail glasses, serve immediately.

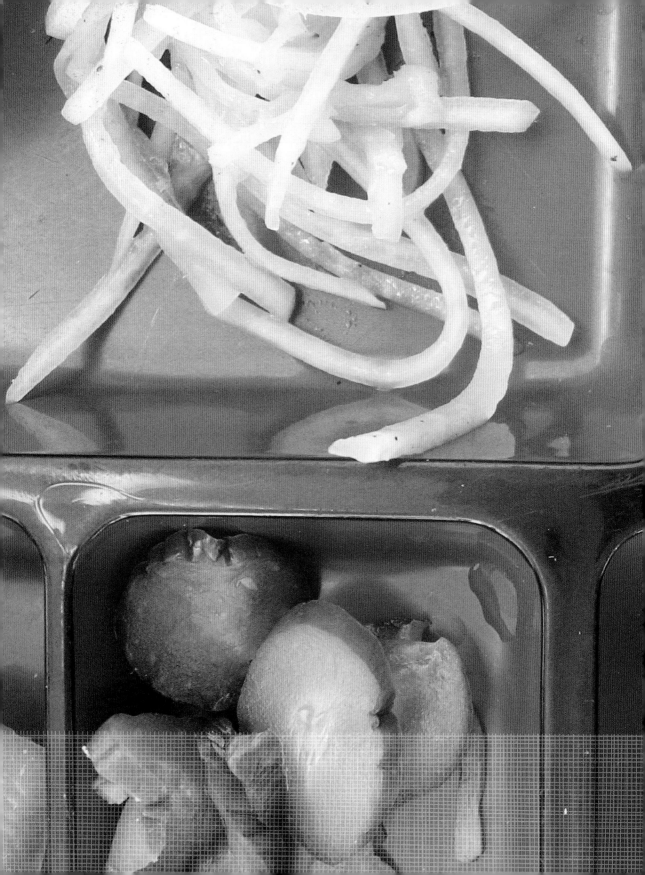

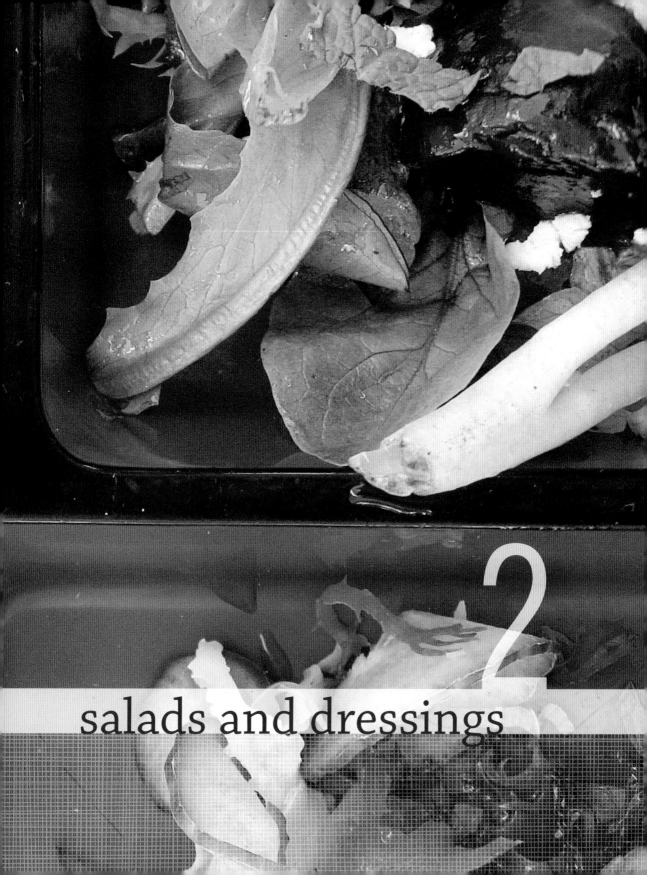

2

salads and dressings

Whole Food Nutrition

Asian cuisine will include ingredients in recipes for their medicinal and superfood value. As in America, fruits, vegetables, nuts, and seeds are packed with vitamins, minerals, and antioxidants that combat free-radical damage, slow down the signs of aging, and boost our immune system. Superfoods boost our overall health and well-being. In Asia, superfoods are known to boost our Qi, the circulating life energy that in Chinese philosophy is inherent in all things. It's our available energy, or life force.

Fruits and vegetables like green mango, papaya, coconut, pineapple, daikon radish, peppers, spinach, and romaine provide enzymes, vitamins, and antioxidants that keep us healthy, plus fiber and structured water that's naturally cleansing, detoxifying, and hydrating. Specifically, coconut, fig, dates, shiitake mushrooms, and squash help tonify our Qi because they release energy steadily into our system over a long period of time.

Many herbs and spices like ginger, chile, lemongrass, Asian lime leaf, basil, mint, and parsley are used medicinally to decrease inflammation, increase circulation, detoxify, cleanse, and boost overall health. And, fermented foods like miso and soy sauce and pickled vegetables like kimchi provide us with valuable probiotics that help build a healthy digestive system (see chapter 3 for more on probiotics).

Black pepper has antiseptic and antioxidant properties. Cardamom helps open the respiratory passages. Cinnamon dries dampness in the body, increases circulation, and aids digestion. Garlic fights infections. Ginger is an antiseptic and anti-inflammatory.

Nuts and seeds like sesame seeds, flax, cashews, and almonds are high in calcium, build strong, healthy bones, and provide vitamins so our skin can build collagen to maintain a youthful complexion and glow. Nuts and seeds, vegetables, and sea vegetables are considered neutral and balanced someplace between opposing yin and yang. Yin and yang describe how seemingly opposite forces are interconnected and dependent upon each other in our natural world. The key is to sit neutral, like these balanced foods: to sit at the center for optimum health and power.

Sea vegetables are known as an ancient Asian longevity secret for their rich minerals, vitamins, iodine, and protein. The minerals found in the ocean are the same as those found in human blood, and sea vegetables are a great source of folate, magnesium, iron, and calcium. Sea vegetables contain lignans, which are plant compounds that protect against cancer. Studies have found diets high in folate-rich foods significantly reduce the risk for colon cancer. Sea vegetables are also high in magnesium, which has been shown to reduce high blood pressure and prevent heart attacks and may help restore normal sleep patterns in menopausal women. Sea vegetables are considered one of the world's healthiest foods because of their rich mineral content and health benefits. To avoid heavy metals from the ocean, choose organic sea vegetables. Most can be purchased dry at natural food markets, Asian markets, or online and reconstituted at home. Sea vegetables are available at www.GoSuperLife.com.

Salads and Dressings

Take a walk down the street in Seoul, South Korea; Bali, Indonesia; or Phuket, Thailand and you'll notice how most sidewalks are filled with fresh produce for sale. Some offerings are brought in from local farms, while others are gathered as wild edibles and weeds from within the city.

I've made it a habit to visit my favorite farmers' market each week to pick up everything that looks good to me. I bring it home and prep most of it immediately. I wash my greens and put together a salad mix. Then, I'll make double and triple batches of dressings and store them in jars in the fridge. This way, I always have salad and dressing ready to go for busy days when I have little time to eat.

Salads are simple and fast to make and work great as sides for entertaining or as a meal on their own. I do include a couple more complex salad recipes in this chapter, which you may find to be more substantial. Me, I just love all these salads on their own, paired with another salad or two, and also served alongside other dishes or in wraps. Each salad ties together the key spices and herbs for fresh Asian flavors. Find whatever works for you and enjoy your greens!

SESAME ROMAINE SALAD

Korea

MAKES 4 SERVINGS

This was a salad I enjoyed almost daily on my last visit to Korea. It's a refreshingly simple and light salad that can be whipped up in no time flat. The dressing, which has a slight barbecue flavor, can be kept in your fridge for several weeks. Consider making a double batch to keep on hand. Adjust to suit your heat and spice levels by using more or less chile pepper. A great add-on to any dish as a side or appetizer.

DRESSING

3 tablespoons toasted sesame oil

1 tablespoon Nama Shoyu, Bragg Liquid Aminos, or tamari

1 tablespoon agave syrup, date syrup, or maple syrup

⅛ teaspoon Korean chile pepper, or cayenne, to taste

SALAD

6 cups bite-size romaine pieces

2 tablespoons sliced white or yellow onion

Place all dressing ingredients into a small bowl or jar and stir or shake to mix.

Place salad ingredients in a large mixing bowl. Toss with dressing.

Serve salad in four serving bowls.

Tossed salad will keep for a day in the fridge. Dressing will keep stored on its own in fridge for a week or longer.

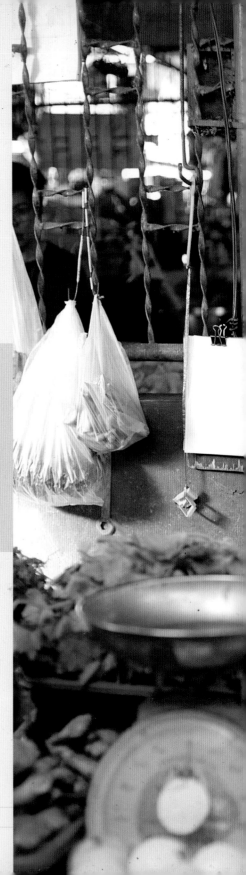

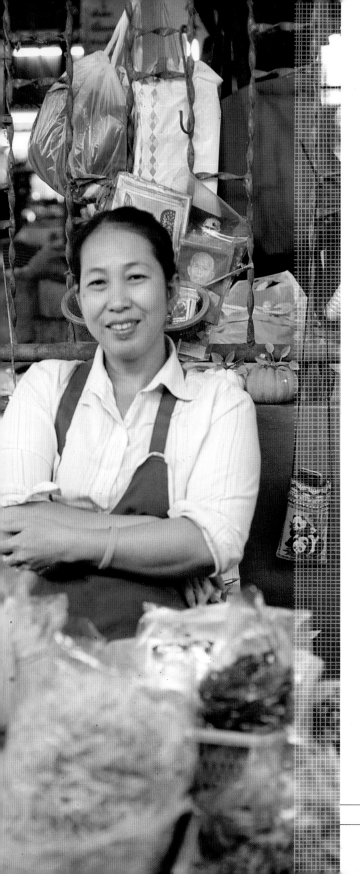

OPEN SESAME

Sesame is high in calcium and there-fore great for building strong teeth and bones and combating osteoporosis. A handful of sesame seeds are said to contain more calcium than a glass of dairy milk. These seeds contain sesa-min and sesamolin, known to prevent the development of and growth of cancer cells and help in cancer treat-ment. Sesame lowers and prevents high blood pressure and high choles-terol and protects against the develop-ment of cardiovascular diseases.

Magnesium in sesame seeds has been shown to help eliminate migraine attacks, headaches, and dizziness and to prevent asthma at-tacks. Packed with vitamin E, sesame helps strengthen our nervous system and builds youthful skin and shiny, strong hair. It helps maintain good di-gestive health, and the fiber prevents constipation.

In Asia, black sesame seeds are said to be so full of vital nutrients that it will restore color back into gray hair.

MISO

Miso is a fermented soybean paste that plays a big role in the northeast Asian diet. It's an all-purpose, high-protein, and high vitamin B-12 seasoning made from soybeans, rice or barley, salt, and a cultured starter called koji. (Koji is to miso what malt is to beer.) The mixture is left to ferment and mature in cedar wood or ceramic vats for as long as five years. I remember seeing ceramic vats buried in the earth for storage in Korea as a child.

The result is a smooth texture similar to a chunky peanut butter that comes in many different colors from a lighter yellow to red to chocolate brown and almost black. Each has its own unique flavor and aroma. The lighter color is usually sweeter and mellower, while the darker is meaty, rich, and more pungent.

Miso has been found to be mentioned in China as early as 200 B.C. where it was known as "chiang." Buddhist monks later brought miso from China to Korea and Japan.

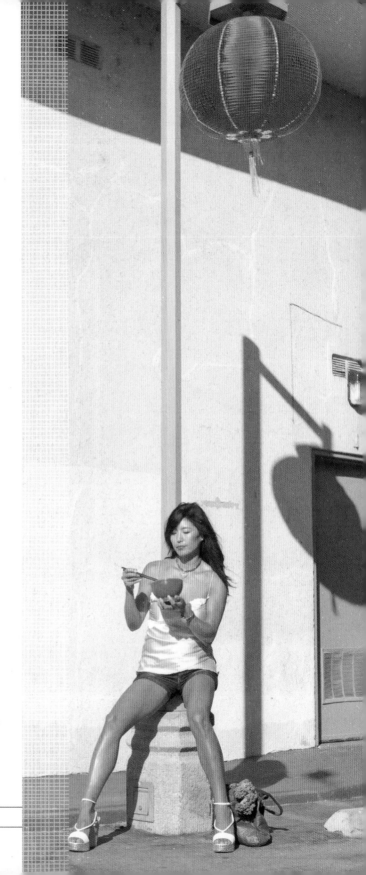

SPINACH WITH KREAMY MISO DRESSING

Japan

MAKES 4 SERVINGS

Miso is a probiotic, fermented, living food that contains many beneficial microorganisms and plays a large part in the Japanese and Korean diet.

This is a quick dressing made by blending celery with miso, olive oil, ginger, and garlic. The celery has natural sodium and adds flavor, texture, and body to the dressing. The flavor of this dressing is so full, all you need for the salad is one ingredient, and the spinach for a creamy green pairs well with a colorful main or secondary dish.

I like to make double batches and keep leftover dressing in a jar in my fridge. This way, I have healthy dressing ready to go for my next salad.

DRESSING

1 cup chopped celery (about 1 stalk)

1 tablespoon miso

1 tablespoon extra-virgin olive oil

½ teaspoon ginger

½ teaspoon garlic

1 to 2 tablespoons filtered water, as needed

Pinch of ground white pepper, optional

SALAD

6 cups spinach

To make dressing, place all ingredients into high-speed blender, adding only enough water for a thick consistency. The water level of your celery will determine how much extra water you will need to add. So add water slowly. Blend smooth.

To serve, place spinach into four serving bowls. Top with dressing and serve.

Dressing will keep for 4 to 5 days in fridge when stored on its own.

VARIATION: *Try the Kreamy Miso Dressing over arugula or a mix of spinach and arugula.*

GREEN MANGO AND COCONUT NOODLE SALAD

Thailand

MAKES 4 SERVINGS

Lemongrass, fresh coconut meat, lime juice, garlic, ginger, and Asian lime leaf give this salad an authentic Thai flavor. Shredded unripe green mango and sweet fresh coconut meat are tossed with a lemongrass and lime juice dressing to make a delicious salad that's beautifully colorful.

Make sure you save the water from your fresh Thai baby coconuts. It's fresh, full of electrolytes, and great served over ice as an accompaniment to this salad, or blended into a smoothie.

DRESSING

½ teaspoon garlic

¼ teaspoon chopped fresh chile pepper or ⅛ teaspoon dried

1 tablespoon chopped lemongrass

1 tablespoon Nama Shoyu, Bragg Liquid Aminos, or tamari

2 teaspoons lime juice

1 tablespoon agave syrup or maple syrup

2 tablespoons chopped cashews

SALAD

1 cup peeled, julienned or shredded green mango, from about 1 whole mango

½ cup sliced into ½-inch wide strips coconut meat

¼ cup shredded carrot (1 small carrot)

¼ cup julienned red bell pepper (⅓ pepper)

1 tablespoon sliced red onion

1 teaspoon chopped scallion

1 teaspoon julienned Asian lime leaf

¼ teaspoon julienned ginger

4 sprigs cilantro for garnish

To make dressing, place garlic, chiles, and lemongrass into a food processor or mortar and pestle. Grind into small pieces. Scoop mixture into large mixing bowl. Add Nama Shoyu, lime juice, agave syrup, and cashews, and stir to mix well.

Shred green mango using a mandoline with the shredding attachment or a handheld vegetable shredder (it looks like a vegetable peeler). Add all salad ingredients to dressing mixture in the large mixing bowl. Toss to mix well.

Arrange on four serving plates. Garnish with a sprig of fresh cilantro.

Will keep for 2 to 3 days in fridge.

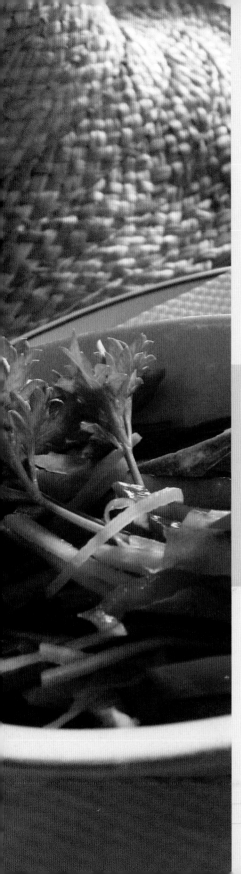

CARROT, CUCUMBER, AND RED BELL PEPPER MATCHSTICK SALAD

Indonesia

MAKES 4 SERVINGS

A classic tri-color julienned salad with a twist of chile spice and tart vinegar that I was introduced to during a month-long visit to Bali, Indonesia. It was served as a side garnish, but I'd order a bowl of it to enjoy as a salad. This recipe has a clean, refreshing flavor plus great mouth feel and bite. A simple, smart, and sophisticated salad that adds vibrant color and taste to any dinner party table and alongside any other dish.

1 cup julienned carrots (about 1 medium carrot)

1 cup julienned cucumbers (about 1 medium cucumber)

1 cup julienned red bell pepper (about 1 whole pepper)

¼ cup thinly sliced red onion (about ½ small onion)

1 teaspoon apple cider vinegar

1 tablespoon extra-virgin olive oil

⅛ to ¼ teaspoon chopped fresh chile pepper, to taste, or a pinch cayenne

¼ teaspoon sea salt

Place ingredients into mixing bowl, and toss to mix.

Serve and enjoy immediately.

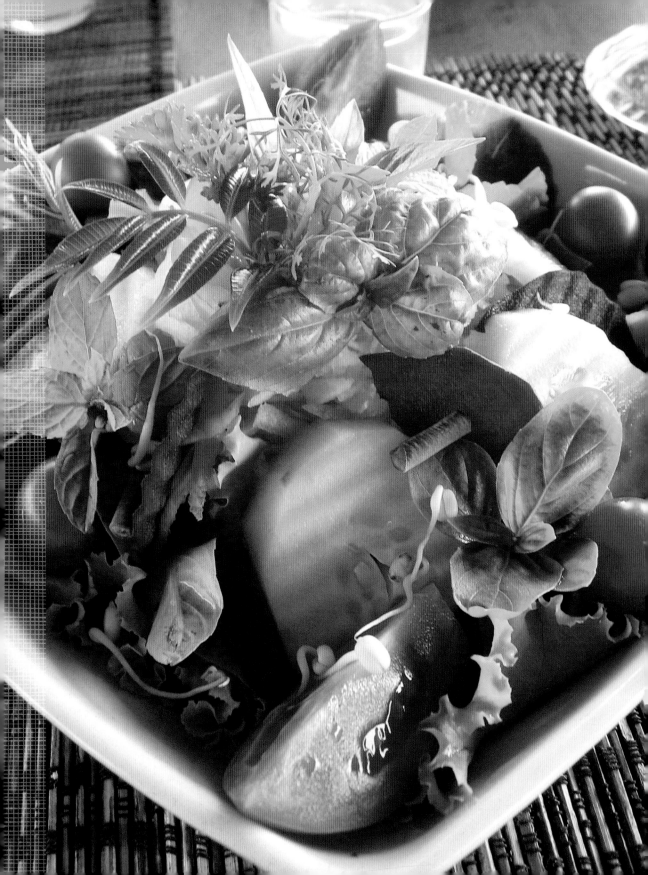

RAINBOW SALAD WITH TAHINI DRESSING

Indonesia

MAKES 4 SERVINGS

A multicolored salad full of textures and flavors from fresh basil and refreshing mint mixed with red beets, carrots, cucumbers, and daikon radish. Tossed in a creamy tahini dressing made with mulled sesame seeds and vitamin C-rich lemon juice.

TAHINI DRESSING (MAKES 1 CUP)

¾ cup tahini

½ cup fresh lemon juice

⅓ cup Bragg Liquid Aminos

⅓ to ½ cup filtered water, as needed to desired consistency

GARNISH

⅓ cup fresh mint, whole leaves

¼ cup fresh basil, whole leaves

SALAD

1 cup cherry tomatoes

½ cup shredded carrot (about 1 medium carrot)

½ cup shredded daikon radish (about ¼ of a small radish)

½ cup mung bean sprouts

½ cup sliced red beets, cut into thin discs (about ½ large beet)

½ cup sliced cucumber (about 1 small cucumber)

4 cups torn and lightly packed green leaf lettuce

Into your blender, place all dressing ingredients. Blend to mix well. Add water as needed for desired texture.

In a large mixing bowl, place tomatoes, carrot, daikon, bean sprouts, beets, and cucumber. Toss with dressing. Add lettuce last, toss lightly to mix.

Serve salad in four bowls and garnish with fresh mint and basil. Enjoy immediately.

Dressing will keep for 5 days in airtight container in fridge. Salad will keep for 3 days when stored separately in fridge.

GREEN PAPAYA SALAD

Thailand

MAKES 4 SERVINGS

Green Papaya Salad is served by most street vendors in Thailand. It's a healthy salad made of shredded papaya seasoned with fresh lime juice, savory garlic, and spicy Thai red chiles. I love spice and like to use a strong chile that's full of kick. But, feel free to adjust the amount of spice to a level that works for you. Since the spiciest part of the chile is in the seeds, consider removing them from your chile pepper to decrease the spice level. And, if you want a mellower garlic flavor, cut down the garlic to ½ teaspoon.

For this recipe, choose an unripe papaya that's green and very firm, so that you'll be able to shred it.

DRESSING

½ teaspoon garlic, to taste

¼ to ½ teaspoon chopped red chile pepper, from about 1 whole Thai red chile, to taste

½ cup chopped green bean, cut into 1¼-inch lengths

1 tablespoon Nama Shoyu, or 1 tablespoon Bragg Liquid Aminos

3 tablespoons lime juice

2 tablespoons agave syrup

2 tablespoons chopped almonds

SALAD

2 cups peeled and shredded green papaya

½ cup shredded carrot (about 1 small carrot)

½ cup shredded green cabbage

½ cup halved cherry tomatoes

GARNISH

¼ cup fresh cilantro leaves

To make dressing, grind garlic and chiles in a food processor or mortar and pestle. Add green beans, and grind into small pieces. Add Nama Shoyu, lime juice, agave syrup, and almonds, and pulse to mix well.

Place salad ingredients in a large mixing bowl. Toss with dressing.

Serve onto four plates and garnish with cilantro leaves.

Dressing will keep for 4 to 5 days in fridge. Salad will keep for 2 days when stored separately. Tossed salad will keep for 1 day in fridge.

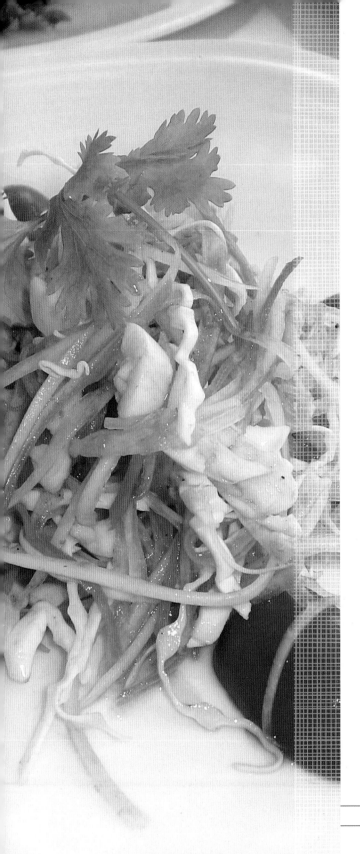

PAPAYA POWER

Green unripe papaya contains a proteolytic enzyme called papain, an excellent digestive aid that's said to digest two hundred times its weight in protein and helps our body's enzymes absorb maximum nutrients from our food. The carbohydrates in papaya are mostly an invert sugar, a predigested food.

Papaya and the papain enzyme have anti-inflammatory properties that reduce inflammation in diseases like rheumatoid arthritis, gout, and asthma. Papain is most concentrated in the skin of an unripe, green papaya; this skin can be used to treat jellyfish stings and other wounds by applying it directly to the injury.

Papain is also a natural laxative, has been found to prevent colon cancer and protect against heart disease.

SEAWEED AND DAIKON SALAD

Korea

MAKES 4 SERVINGS

A simple salad of mineral- and protein-rich wakame sea vegetable and fresh daikon, massaged with a sweet and tart soy and sesame dressing. Korean food preparation uses our hands to massage sauces and dressings into our vegetables, rather than tossing with utensils, as in this recipe. Feel free to use your bare hands, after washing well, or you can wear a plastic or latex glove, disposable or reusable. Reusable is always more eco (environmentally friendly), of course.

Note: Dried wakame will grow about three times in volume once hydrated. To hydrate your wakame, place it in a bowl with about three times the amount of water as wakame, and set aside for about 10 to 15 minutes to reconstitute. Squeeze out excess liquid before using in this recipe. Also note that Korean chile powder is milder than cayenne. So use much less cayenne if substituting. Gradually add more, and keep tasting to avoid making this dish too spicy.

DRESSING

2 tablespoons Nama Shoyu or tamari

3 tablespoons agave, maple syrup, or brown rice syrup

2 tablespoons apple cider vinegar

½ tablespoon minced garlic

½ tablespoon Korean chile powder, or ⅛ teaspoon cayenne, to taste

1 tablespoon toasted sesame oil

SALAD

1 cup dried wakame, hydrate by soaking in 3 cups water for 10 minutes, squeeze out excess liquid before using

½ cup julienned daikon radish

GARNISH

½ tablespoon sesame seeds

Whisk together all dressing ingredients in a large mixing bowl. Add wakame and daikon to bowl and use your hands to massage and mix well.

To serve, portion salad into four bowls and sprinkle with sesame seeds as garnish.

Will keep for 2 to 3 days in fridge.

RADISH SPROUT AND PEA SALAD WITH PARSLEY DRESSING

Korea

MAKES 4 SERVINGS

In its most authentic form, this salad calls for cooked edamame (green soybeans). As with any legume, raw soybeans are toxic and don't taste very good, either. I use fresh peas instead, with cucumbers, carrots, iceberg lettuce, and spicy radish sprouts for a crispy cool salad served with a blended apple and parsley dressing.

Radish sprouts are germinated radish seeds that have just started to grow small leaves; they have a peppery flavor like radish. As with all sprouts, radish sprouts are high in vitamins A, B, C, E, and K, as well as zinc, calcium, and iron. To avoid harmful bacteria passed during food handling of sprouts, I prefer to grow my own when possible. To grow your own sprouts, see page 32.

DRESSING	SALAD
⅓ cup lightly packed parsley	3 cups torn pieces of iceberg lettuce
1 cup peeled, seeded, diced apple (1 medium apple)	½ cup grated carrots (about 1 small carrot)
⅓ cup apple cider vinegar	1 cup julienned cucumbers (about 1 small cucumber)
½ cup extra-virgin olive oil	½ cup radish sprouts
1 tablespoon agave syrup	½ cup peas
⅛ teaspoon sea salt	

Place dressing ingredients into blender. Blend smooth.

To make salad, place lettuce, carrot, and cucumber into a mixing bowl and toss. Transfer to serving bowl and top with radish sprouts and peas.

Serve salad with dressing on the side.

Dressing will keep for 4 days in fridge. Tossed salad will keep for 1 day in fridge.

PINEAPPLE, RED CABBAGE, AND CORN SALAD

Indonesia

MAKES 4 SERVINGS

A refreshing sweet and tart salad made with pineapple, lettuce, corn, and tomato tossed in a light vinaigrette. I use pineapple that is a bit less ripe for a distinct grassy sharpness. If you like a sweeter flavor, choose a riper pineapple.

DRESSING

2 tablespoons extra-virgin olive oil

1 teaspoon apple cider vinegar

2 teaspoons agave syrup

¼ teaspoon sea salt

A pinch or 2 of black pepper, to taste

SALAD

2 cups torn red leaf lettuce

1 cup shredded red cabbage

1 cup diced pineapple

½ cup tomato wedges (about 1 small tomato)

½ cup corn kernels

¼ cup thinly sliced yellow onion rings (about ¼ small onion)

To make dressing, whisk all ingredients together in a small bowl or jar.

Place all salad ingredients into mixing bowl. Toss with dressing to mix.

To serve, portion onto four serving bowls or plates. Enjoy immediately.

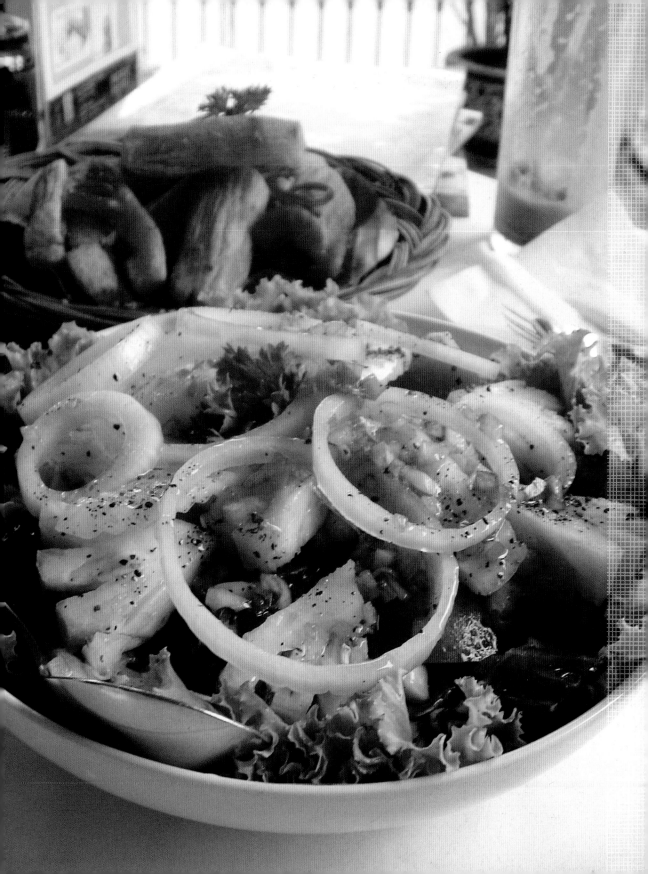

HUNGRY FOR PROTEIN

When I was younger, I didn't worry about my protein intake. Today, my tune has changed, and I realize our bodies need more protein, especially as we age.

Protein is the building block for collagen in our skin, the matrix keeping our skin taught, elastic, moist, and supple. Protein builds lean muscle mass and keeps our metabolism buzzing.

Great sources of protein include dark leafy greens; sea vegetables like nori, arame, dulse, kelp, spirulina; wheatgrass juice; and nuts and seeds like hemp protein and buckwheat groats.

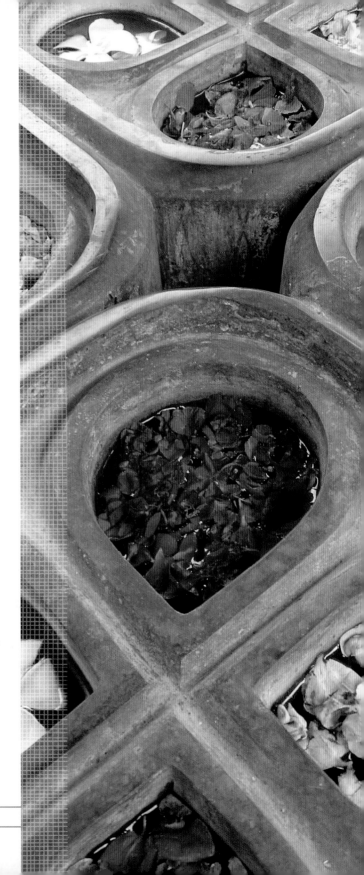

ARAME AND NORI SALAD WITH MICRO GREENS AND CABBAGE

Japan

MAKES 4 SERVINGS

I make sure to keep dry sea vegetables stocked in my kitchen always. They're a great source of minerals from the ocean and protein, and I love adding them to my salads.

Arame is a type of kelp that's high in calcium, iodine, iron, magnesium, and vitamin A, plus other minerals. Purchase it dry and reconstitute it in just 10 minutes by soaking it in filtered water. Nori comes in sheets and is most commonly used to wrap rice into rolls with vegetables. Nori is another sea vegetable high in minerals, iodine, and protein. I use micro greens in this recipe. They're tiny edible greens from the seeds of vegetables, herbs, or other plants. They are between 1 and 2 inches long and have much more developed flavors, colors, and texture than sprouts. Micro greens are different from sprouts in that sprouts don't need sunlight to grow, but micro greens do. Micro greens also grow four or more leaves.

SALAD
1½ cups dried arame

1 cup shredded green cabbage

1 cup micro greens

2 sheets nori, torn into bite-size pieces

GARNISH
2 tablespoons chopped scallions

DRESSING
2 teaspoons toasted sesame oil

1 teaspoon apple cider vinegar

¼ teaspoon grated ginger

⅛ teaspoon sea salt, to taste

Soak arame in 2 cups of water. Set aside for 10 minutes or longer to hydrate. Squeeze to remove excess liquid before using.

Thinly slice cabbage with a mandoline slicer or a knife. In mixing bowl, add cabbage, micro greens, and nori.

Next, add dressing ingredients to the bowl and toss to mix well. Add arame mixture and toss to mix well.

To serve, top with scallions and enjoy.

Will keep for 1 day in fridge.

BLACK AND TAN ENCRUSTED COCONUT MEAT ON A BED OF SHREDDED DAIKON, CARROTS, AND CUCUMBERS TOSSED IN GODDESS DRESSING

Japan

MAKES 4 SERVINGS

Thai baby coconut meat is coated in black and tan sesame seeds, then dehydrated into a jerky texture to create a beautiful color and presentation. If you can't find black sesame seeds, you can always just use tan, and if you want to create the black-and-tan look, try adding in a few poppy seeds instead. Placed on top of shredded daikon radish, red bell pepper, carrots, and cucumbers, Black and Tan Encrusted Coconut Meat is a beautiful complement to any dish. I recommend making double or triple the batch, so you have extra on hand for the next meal.

If you don't have a dehydrator yet, you can use your oven on the lowest setting to dry your coconut meat. To keep it as raw as possible, prop the oven door open using a chopstick. Hardly eco green, but hopefully you'll be inspired to acquire a dehydrator.

BLACK AND TAN ENCRUSTED COCONUT MEAT

2 cups Thai baby coconut meat (keep pieces as large as possible) from about 3 to 4 Thai baby coconuts

2 tablespoons Nama Shoyu or Bragg Liquid Aminos

2 tablespoons extra-virgin olive oil

½ cup crushed tan and/or black sesame seeds

SALAD

2 cups shredded daikon radish (about ½ small radish)

½ cup sliced carrot (sliced into circles, about 1 small carrot)

¼ cup cucumbers (sliced into circles, about 1 small cucumber)

¼ cup julienned baby red bell pepper (about ¼ red pepper)

DRESSING

½ teaspoon minced garlic

½ teaspoon sea salt

½ cup tahini

1 tablespoon Nama Shoyu

1½ tablespoons apple cider vinegar

2 teaspoons agave syrup

⅓ cup water, as needed

2 tablespoons chopped fresh parsley

To make coconut meat, toss coconut with Nama Shoyu and olive oil. Crush sesame seeds using a mortar and pestle. Spread sesame onto a small plate or bowl and dip each piece of coconut meat into sesame, then place on dehydrator trays. Dry at 104°F for 6 to 8 hours.

To make dressing, mash garlic and salt into a paste in a small bowl or a mortar and pestle. Add tahini, Nama Shoyu, vinegar, agave syrup, and mix well. Add just enough water gradually (a teaspoon at a time) to desired consistency. Stir in parsley. Place salad ingredients into large mixing bowl. Add dressing, and toss to mix well.

Serve by placing salad onto four plates. Top with dehydrated, sesame-encrusted coconut meat.

Black and Tan Encrusted Coconut Meat will keep at room temperature for several days and even longer when dehydrated more. Dressing will keep for 4 to 5 days in fridge.

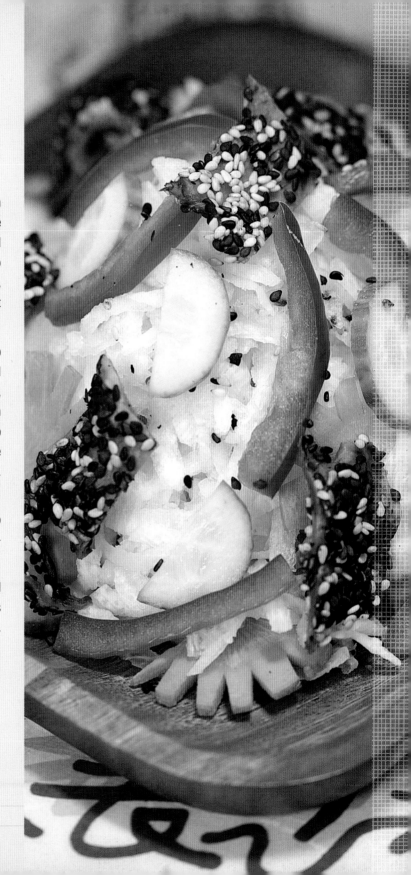

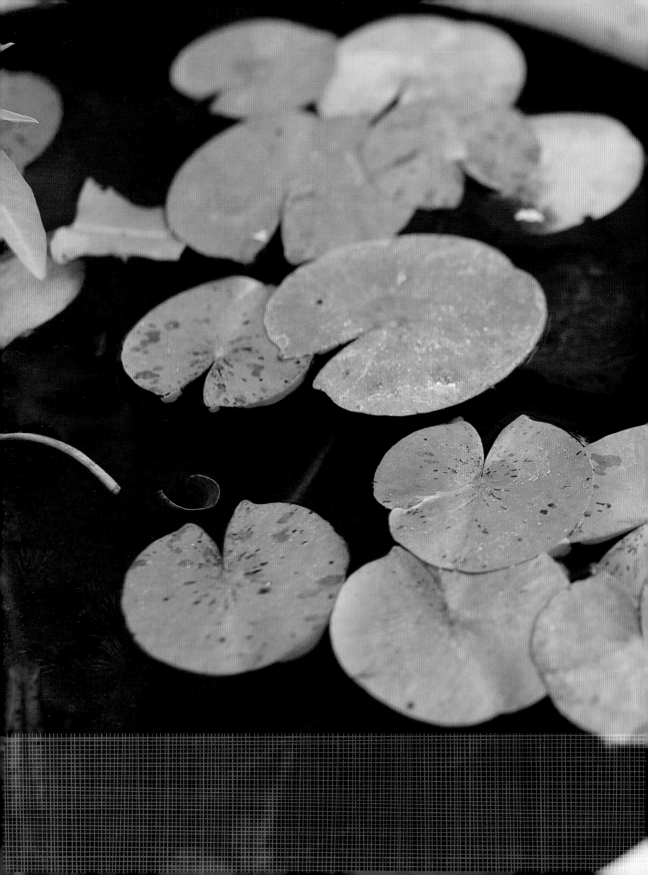

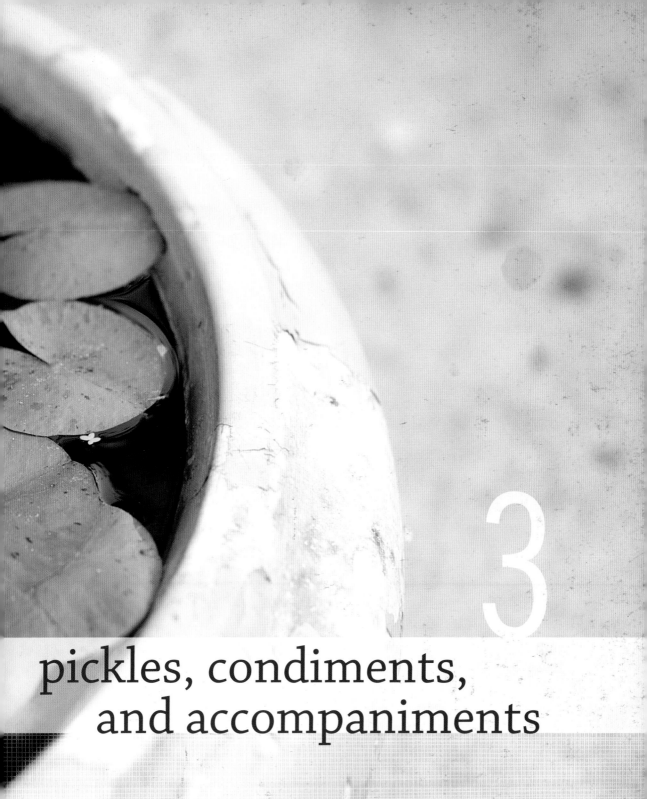

3

pickles, condiments, and accompaniments

Probiotics

Probiotic foods are quickly becoming the latest healthy living trend. They're friendly bacteria that aid our digestion so we can better absorb nutrients from our food. The easier it is for us to digest, the less energy we need to expend to break food down in our belly, and the more energy we have remaining. They also help with healthy elimination of waste from our bodies and are detoxifying. Other breakthrough discoveries on the benefits of probiotics include enhanced immune function, decreased inflammation, prevention of allergies and asthma, elimination of yeast infections, and improvement in overall health.

Antibiotics are a powerful drug we love to use in America to treat infections caused by micro-organisms. Unfortunately, antibiotics kill all bacteria, good and bad. So it's extremely important to restore our body's natural balance of healthy bacteria by eating fermented pickled foods and drinking cultured drinks.

One great way to enjoy probiotics is by eating pickled vegetables like Korean kimchi. I include three cultured, easy kimchi recipes made using cabbage, daikon radish, and cucumber. Three fast pickles and eight recipes for Korean-inspired marinated vegetable dishes called *namul* are included, too. Namuls are great side dishes and make for a delicious add-on to any recipe.

For more on fermented drinks like kombucha, kefir, and rejuvelac, as well as more pickled vegetable recipes, check out my previous book, *Ani's Raw Food Essentials*.

Pickles

Serve pickles with any dish for a tangy accompaniment, additional texture, and more flavor. Adding pickles to a dish bumps up its complexity and level of sophistication. Some of these pickles can be enjoyed immediately, while the other, more probiotic rich pickles will take about 3 days to ferment.

In fermentation, metal of all sorts, as in bowls and utensils, should be avoided because they interact and damage probiotic activity. In Korea, vegetables are pickled in ceramic, and it's thought that the ceramic, over time, seeps with flavor to create a rich, aged taste. Vegetables should be marinated in a bowl, and covered lightly, if at all. To pickle, transfer into a glass jar or ceramic container a leav om temperature in a dark place until desired flavor.

CUCUMBER PICKLE
Indonesia

MAKES 2 CUPS

PICKLING TIME: IMMEDIATE

A simple, quick, and delish pickle made with cucumber semi-circles, seasoned with tart vinegar, fresh lemongrass, onion, and spicy chile.

2 cups sliced cucumbers (cut in semi-circles, about 2 medium cucumbers)

1 teaspoon apple cider vinegar

1 teaspoon minced lemongrass

1 teaspoon chopped red onion

⅛ to ¼ teaspoon chopped red chile, to taste

Place all ingredients into mixing bowl. Toss to mix well.

Enjoy immediately, or store in airtight container in fridge for 3 to 4 days.

FAST CUCUMBER SALAD
Thailand

MAKES 2 CUPS

PICKLING TIME: 30 MINUTES

This tangy sweet cucumber pickle takes only a few minutes to prepare, another 30 minutes to marinate, and should be enjoyed immediately.

2 cups thinly sliced cucumbers (about 2 cucumbers)

¾ cup thinly sliced red onion (about 1 small onion)

2 teaspoons agave syrup or maple syrup

2 teaspoons sea salt

¼ cup apple cider vinegar

Place all ingredients into mixing bowl, and toss to mix well. Set aside for 30 minutes to marinate. Serve and enjoy immediately.

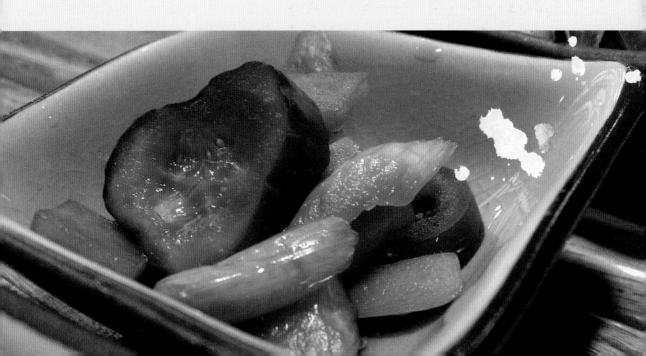

DAIKON LEMON PICKLE

Japan

MAKES 2 CUPS

PICKLING TIME: 1 HOUR

Daikon is a really large white radish that's popular in both Korea and Japan. It grows in the winter and can be found at natural food stores and Asian markets.

This is a tart, cool pickle that works well as a companion to spicy dishes.

2 cups peeled and very thinly sliced daikon (about 1½ pounds radish)

3 tablespoons sea salt

BRINE

1 teaspoon toasted sesame oil

1 tablespoon agave syrup or maple syrup

1 tablespoon apple cider vinegar

⅓ cup lemon juice

½ teaspoon minced garlic

1 teaspoon lemon zest

In a large colander set over a bowl, place sliced daikon. Use your hands to toss with salt. Set aside for 15 minutes to release water. In large mixing bowl, whisk together all brine ingredients. Set aside.

Rinse daikon under running water to remove salt. Squeeze to remove excess liquid. Add to brine in mixing bowl and coat well. Set aside to marinate for 1 hour.

Enjoy immediately, or refrigerate in airtight container for several weeks.

CRUNCHY CUCUMBER SLICES

Korea

MAKES 2 CUPS

PICKLING TIME: IMMEDIATELY

This crunchy pickle is called *oi jih* in Korean. Cucumber slices are tossed in sea salt to soften and are then squeezed to completely remove all excess liquid. The crisp slices are tossed in toasted sesame oil for flavor (you can use raw if preferred), savory garlic, chile powder, and a touch of sweetener.

2 pickling cucumbers, or smaller cucumbers, sliced into rounds

2 tablespoons sea salt

½ tablespoon minced garlic

1 tablespoon toasted sesame oil

1 tablespoon Korean chile powder, or ¼ teaspoon cayenne, to taste

1 tablespoon agave or brown rice syrup

½ tablespoon sesame seeds

½ tablespoon sliced scallion (green part only, for color)

Toss cucumber slices in salt and set aside for 15 minutes to release liquid. Then, completely squeeze all the liquid out of the slices. Place into a bowl and add garlic, sesame oil, chile powder, and agave syrup and toss to mix well.

To serve, top with sesame seeds and scallion.

Will keep for a week or longer in fridge.

INCLUDING, NOT EXCLUDING

I encourage including more nutrient-dense foods into any diet. The way I look at it, if I'm going to eat calories and place wear and tear on my body to digest food, I want to make sure that food is full of the vitamins, minerals, and enzymes my body needs to perform and stay healthy. As we eat more nutrient-rich foods, we naturally have less room in our belly for less beneficial food. The healthy foods effortlessly elbow out less healthy options.

This idea of inclusion can extend beyond just food and into the way we think about life, love, and business. In business, it's more fun for me to think in terms of building playgrounds where people can come and work, share, and play together. That's more fun than building a battlefield where someone has to lose for another to win. I believe in win-win situations where those involved gain more by working together than alone.

This inclusive ideal is typical of the traditional Asian lifestyle. Opposite from the American "me" culture, Asian culture is about putting the good of the community above one's selfish desires. With this community view it becomes easier to choose decisions that won't damage our environment or harm other people and beings. We are all connected, so harming another means harming one's self.

These days, we're driven to accumulate financial wealth, and it doesn't seem to matter what we do to get it. In the Asian tradition, more value is placed on things that money can't buy. Happiness, family, community, wellness, health, respect, manners, age, wisdom, and honor are desired and held in high regard. As our world grows smaller and East and West merge, it's important to find the healthy balance between all the great things both cultures have to offer.

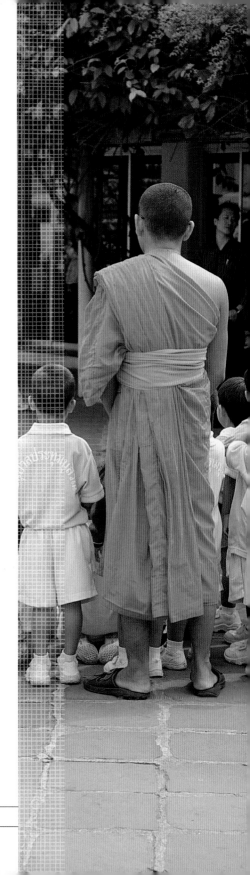

EASY KIMCHI

Korea

MAKES 1½ PINTS

PICKLING TIME: 3 DAYS

I introduce several kimchi recipes in *Ani's Raw Food Essentials*; here's an easy one to get you started. You'll need two 2-quart jars for the pickling here; you can find these at natural food stores or reuse containers from other foods.

1 large head of napa cabbage, cored and chopped into 2-inch pieces

⅓ cup sea salt

2 teaspoons minced garlic

1 tablespoon grated ginger

1 teaspoon Korean chile flakes or cayenne powder

¼ cup sliced scallion

Into a large colander placed over a bowl, put chopped cabbage. Use your hands to toss with salt. Set aside 45 minutes to release water and wilt.

Next, rinse excess salt from cabbage under running water. Squeeze excess liquid from cabbage and place it into a large, clean mixing bowl. Add remaining ingredients and use a spoon to toss and mix well.

Pack into two 2-quart glass jars and press firmly until juices come up to the top and cover the cabbage. Leave at least 1 inch of air at top of jar. Cover tightly and let the jars sit at room temperature for 3 days. The flavor becomes stronger and more fermented the longer the jars sit. Liquid will be released, and the scent will become pungent.

Store kimchi packed down tightly in the jars. Make sure the kimchi is covered with the juice in the jar to keep it fresh. Otherwise, exposed parts can grow mold. Will keep for a month or longer in the fridge.

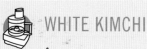

WHITE KIMCHI

Korea

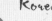

MAKES ABOUT 2 PINTS

PICKLING TIME: 36 HOURS

A kimchi without chile is called White Kimchi. It's popular during the hot summer months as a refreshing pickle on its own and alongside any dish as an accompaniment.

SALT BATH

6 cups filtered water

6 tablespoons coarse sea salt

1 head napa cabbage, cut into 4 quarters lengthwise

FILLING

½ daikon radish, julienned

2 tablespoons coarse salt

¼ cup sliced chives (cut into 2-inch strips)

BRINE

10 cups water

⅓ cup agave or honey or rice syrup

⅓ cup coarse sea salt

FLAVORINGS

1 Asian pear, peeled, seeded, and cubed

½ white onion, diced

7 cloves garlic

1 tablespoon minced ginger

First, make salt bath by mixing the water and salt in a large bowl. Stir to dissolve salt. Add cabbage, cut side up. Put heavy plate on top of cabbage stacked with more plates to weigh down cabbage so it's completely submerged in the salt bath. Set aside 10 to 12 hours at room temperature to soften. When ready to use, drain cabbage, discard salt water, and rinse cabbage with water. Set aside.

Next, make the filling by placing daikon in a large bowl. Sprinkle with salt and set aside to marinate and soften for 20 minutes until water releases. Add chives and toss.

Now, make brine by placing the water, agave syrup, and salt into a large bowl. Mix to dissolve salt, and set aside.

To make flavorings, place the pear, onion, garlic, and ginger into food processor, and process well. Spoon the puree into a nut mylk bag or cheesecloth and then squeeze to catch the juice in a bowl. Add flavorings juice to the large bowl of brine. Discard pulp.

Stuff your softened cabbage with filling mixture by lifting each leaf and distributing some of the radish mix between each leaf (about 1 to 2 tablespoons). This is an optional step, but after all layers have been filled, take the outermost and greenest cabbage leaf and use it to wrap up each quarter into a parcel.

Place stuffed quarters into the large bowl with brine, and submerge fully by placing plates on top of the cabbage to weigh it down. Set aside at room temperature for 24 hours. Transfer to container and refrigerate the kimchi, taking care that it is always completely submerged in the brine, for up to three weeks.

To serve, lift cabbage from brine, and cut crosswise into 2-inch slices across the spine and serve.

Will keep for up to three weeks stored in fridge and fully submerged in brine.

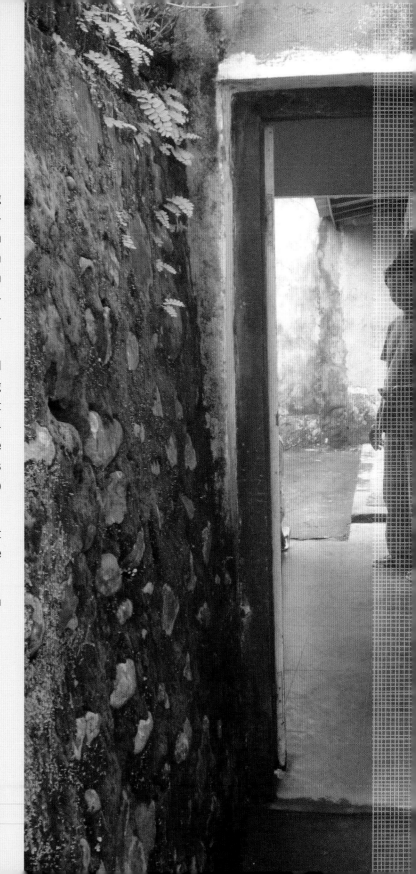

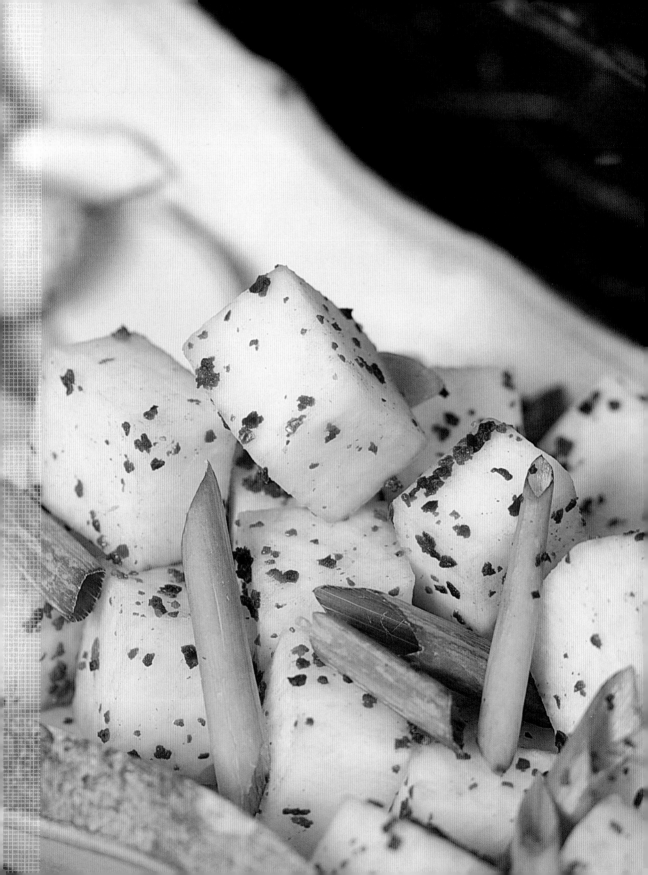

DAIKON KIMCHI

Korea

MAKES ABOUT 2 QUARTS, OR ½ GALLON

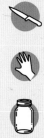

PICKLING TIME: 3 TO 4 DAYS

For better flavor, ideally, you'll want to use a Korean radish. Korean radish is also known as *tae baek* or *moo* in Korean. It's large, about 6 inches long, and has a green tip. It's found in China and Thailand, as well as in Korea. Look for it in Asian grocery stores, or buy seeds and grow your own.

Korean radish is slightly different from daikon. It's stubbier and more round, while the daikon is longer. Daikon is more common, so you can use daikon instead.

1 teaspoon minced garlic

1 tablespoon grated ginger

½ tablespoon Korean chile powder or ½ teaspoon cayenne powder, to taste

½ tablespoon sea salt

½ tablespoon agave syrup

8 cups of cubed daikon radish, from about ½ large daikon radish, peeled and cut into 1-inch cubes

½ cup sliced scallion, cut in 1-inch lengths

In a food processor, or using a mortar and pestle, mince or grind together garlic, ginger, chile powder, and salt. Add agave syrup, mix well, to a paste-like consistency.

Place radish and scallion into a mixing bowl. Wearing gloves, coat daikon evenly with the garlic mixture.

Pack radish into a ½-gallon glass jar, or two 1-quart mason jars, and seal the lid tightly. Set jar in cool, dark cabinet for 3 to 4 days to pickle and ferment.

Refrigerate after opening. Will keep for a couple weeks in fridge.

CUCUMBER KIMCHI

Korea

MAKES ABOUT ½ GALLON

PICKLING TIME: 2 TO 3 DAYS

Cooling cucumbers seasoned with spicy chile make for a dish that's a popular summertime dish in Korea but great all year around. The cucumbers will have a sour flavor plus they absorb all the flavors of garlic, onion, and chile.

CUCUMBERS

10 pickling cucumbers, about 1 pound, slice lengthwise into quarters

⅓ cup sea salt

4 cups filtered water

SPICES

6 cloves garlic, minced

⅓ cup diced yellow onion (about ½ a medium onion)

5 scallions, cut into 1-inch lengths

⅓ cup Korean chile powder, or cayenne

1 tablespoon coarse sea salt

Place cucumbers into large mixing bowl. In another bowl, whisk to dissolve salt into water. Pour over cucumbers. Set aside for 20 to 30 minutes to marinate.

In a large mixing bowl, combine all spice ingredients. Mix well.

Strain cucumbers and lightly rinse with filtered water. Add cucumbers to spice mixture. Mix and coat cucumbers evenly with spices. Transfer cucumbers into a ½-gallon jar, pressing firmly to fill. Close lid tightly.

Set in cool, dark cabinet for 2 to 3 days before opening.

Keep in fridge after opening. Will keep for about 10 days.

Namuls

Namul is a seasoned vegetable side dish, served with rice, that accompanies the majority of most meals in Korea. Namuls are quick to make and are seasoned and mixed, or massaged, by hand with sesame oil, vinegar, chile powder, and sesame seeds. They are also referred to as *moo chim*, which means "massage." You can massage and mix with your bare hands, wear disposable plastic or latex gloves, or better yet, wear rubber gloves that can be washed and reused for the least impact on our planet.

Another name for side dishes in Korean food is *ban chan*. In Korea, the main dish is the rice, and all these namuls, or *ban chan*, are side dishes that accompany the rice. They are usually a bit salty and spicy to add flavor to bland rice. These recipes are delicious on their own, and since I'm not eating these with a starchy cooked rice, I cut back on the saltiness in my recipes.

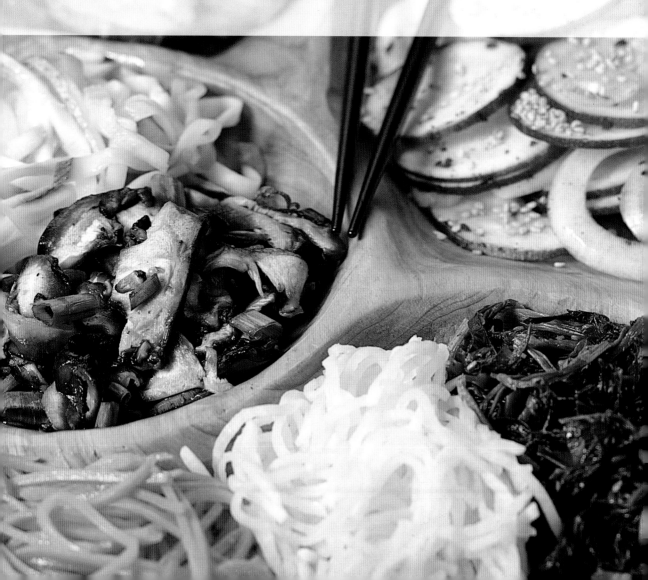

ASPARAGUS NAMUL

Korea

SERVES 4 AS SIDE DISH

Asparagus is marinated in vinegar, soy sauce, sesame oil, garlic, and chile with your bare hands or with gloves on. This dish can be eaten immediately, or set aside to soften for 30 minutes. If you want to soften your asparagus even more, place sliced asparagus in your dehydrator at 104 degrees for a couple of hours to help wilt them before using.

2 cups sliced asparagus, cut diagonally into ¾-inch lengths

1 tablespoon apple cider vinegar

1 tablespoon Nama Shoyu

2 teaspoons sesame seeds

1 teaspoon toasted sesame oil

½ teaspoon minced garlic

⅛ teaspoon Korean chile flakes, or red chile flakes, to taste

Place all ingredients into mixing bowl. Use your hands (you can wear gloves if you prefer) to coat the asparagus and mix well.

Serve immediately or set aside to marinate and allow the asparagus to wilt and soften for 20 to 30 minutes before serving.

Will keep for 2 days in fridge.

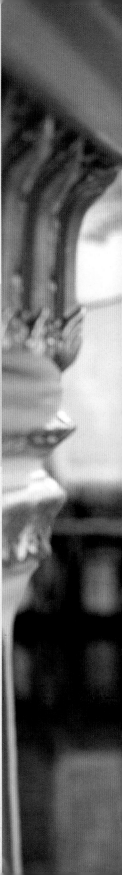

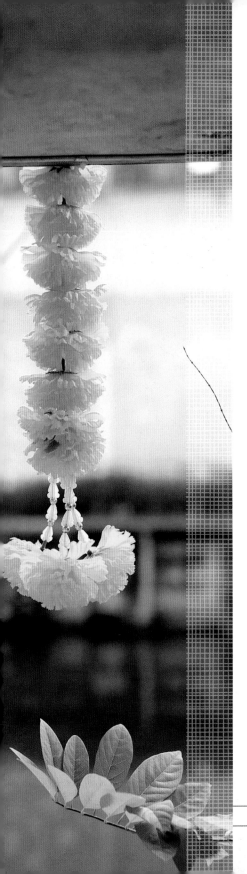

TOASTED SESAME OIL

Toasted sesame oil is what gives many Asian dishes their distinct, nutty flavor. It's obviously cooked, but since I'm using only a tablespoon at a time, I choose to go for the rich flavor. You can always use raw, untoasted oil if you prefer, but the flavor will be milder.

Sesame oil is very high in linoleic acid, which is one of the two essential fatty acids (EFA's) our body is unable to produce. EFA's build healthy blood, arteries, and nerves. They keep skin and other tissues youthful, moist, supple, and healthy. EFAs help regulate blood pressure and cholesterol metabolism and help move biochemicals across cell membranes.

Food processing, including oil and grain refinement, have caused an increase in EFA deficiencies in America. Signs of linoleic acid deficiencies include hair loss, breakouts, mood swings, infections, slow or failed healing of wounds, and in extreme cases, heart, liver, and kidney disease.

Sesame oil is high in vitamin E, an antioxidant that lowers cholesterol levels, and contains magnesium, copper, calcium, iron, zinc, and vitamin B6. These antioxidants slow the aging process and promote longevity. Sesame oil is thought to mitigate anxiety, nerve and bone disorders, and poor circulation. It raises immunity, relieves fatigue and insomnia, promotes strength and vitality, and improves blood circulation.

Sesame oil is used in India for massaging. And, applying it to your hair is said to darken hair color and help prevent hair loss. (see Indian Head Massage, page 142)

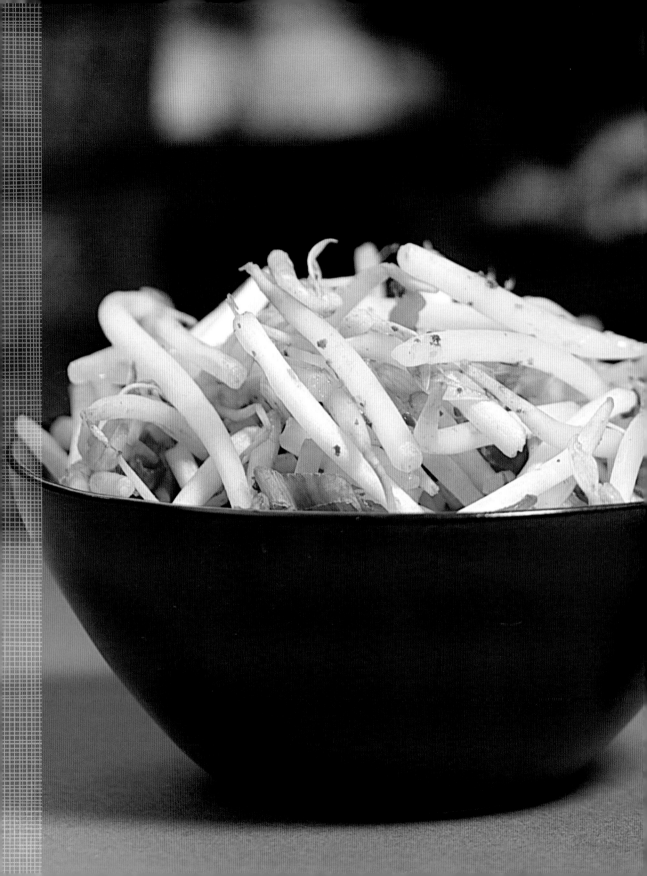

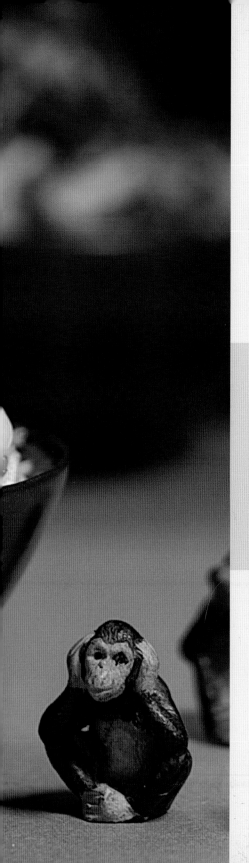

MUNG BEAN SPROUT NAMUL

Korea

SERVES 4 AS SIDE DISH

A simple, fresh way to prepare nutritious mung bean sprouts. It's one of the most popular vegetable side dishes in Korea. Add it to wraps, sprinkle on salads, and serve with any main dish.

In Korea, to minimize the smell of mung bean sprouts, a dash of ginger juice is used. In my recipe, I use julienned ginger instead. But you can use a dash of ginger juice if you prefer.

4 cups bean sprouts

2 tablespoons apple cider vinegar

2 tablespoons toasted sesame oil

1½ teaspoons sea salt

1 teaspoon agave syrup

½ teaspoon minced garlic

¼ teaspoon chile flakes, to taste

1 tablespoon finely chopped scallion

1 teaspoon julienned ginger

Place all ingredients into mixing bowl. Use your hands (you can wear gloves if you prefer) to mix well.

Serve immediately or set aside for 20 to 30 minutes or more until sprouts marinate and soften. Will keep for 2 to 3 days in fridge.

OKRA NAMUL

Korea

SERVES 4 AS SIDE DISH

Okra is a deliciously gooey (okay, slimy) vegetable that I love. A lot of people don't like okra's texture; the gooeyness increases when cooked with water, so eating it raw is less slimy. If you don't like the texture of okra when it's cooked, this recipe may help you change your mind, since it's less slimy. But the slippery nature of okra is intrinsic to the vegetable, giving it a unique texture I love.

3 cups sliced okra (about 12 whole)

2 teaspoons crushed sesame seeds

2 teaspoons toasted sesame oil

¼ teaspoon Korean chile flakes

1 teaspoon apple cider vinegar

2 teaspoons Nama Shoyu

Place all ingredients into a mixing bowl. Use your hands (you can wear gloves if you prefer) to mix well. Set aside for 20 to 30 minutes to marinate and soften.

To serve, transfer into serving bowl.

Will keep for 2 days in fridge.

ZUCCHINI NAMUL

Korea

SERVES 4 AS SIDE DISH

Zucchini marinates and softens resulting in a texture that's very similar to when it's cooked. Flavored with sesame, chile, and onion, this simple namul tastes great in wraps and added to most dishes.

3 cups sliced zucchini, (seeded with a spoon and cut into thin rounds, about 2 medium zucchini)

2 teaspoons toasted sesame oil

2 teaspoons minced yellow onion

1 tablespoon sesame seeds

¼ teaspoon red chile flakes

¼ teaspoon sea salt

Place all ingredients into a mixing bowl. Use your hands (you can wear gloves if you prefer) to mix well.

Serve immediately, or set aside to marinate and soften for 20 minutes before serving.

Will keep for 1 day in fridge.

CUCUMBER NAMUL

Korea

SERVES 4 AS SIDE DISH

A cool and refreshing cucumber side dish with a hint of spice from chile flakes. If you can't find Korean chile flakes, use the traditional flakes we use to sprinkle over cooked pizza. Keep in mind, the pizza chile flakes are spicier, so use less, starting at ⅓ or ½ the amount of the Korean chili, and adjust to taste. I prefer using toasted sesame oil for flavor, but if you want to substitute it with the same amount of raw sesame oil, you can do that, too.

3 cups thinly sliced cucumbers (about 3 whole cucumbers)

1 teaspoon sea salt

1 tablespoon crushed sesame seeds

2 teaspoons toasted sesame oil

2 teaspoons apple cider vinegar

1 teaspoon finely chopped scallion

1 teaspoon agave syrup

¼ teaspoon minced garlic

¼ teaspoon Korean chile flakes, to taste

In a bowl, place cucumber slices and sprinkle with salt. Set aside for 30 minutes to soften and release water. Squeeze out excess liquid by hand. Place cucumbers into a clean mixing bowl with remaining ingredients. Use your hands (you can wear gloves if you prefer) to mix well.

Serve immediately.

Will keep for 1 day in fridge.

SPINACH NAMUL

Korea

SERVES 4 AS SIDE DISH

This is one of my favorite namuls and is one of the most common, along with the mung bean sprout namul. It's similar to a pressed spinach salad and has a similar texture as when blanched. Spinach is tossed with a toasted sesame seed oil for a rich, nutty flavor. It you prefer raw, just use the same amount of raw sesame oil instead.

4 cups packed spinach, washed well and dried, from about 1 bunch

2 teaspoons Nama Shoyu

2 teaspoons toasted sesame oil

½ teaspoon minced garlic

1 tablespoon sliced scallion

1 teaspoon sesame seeds

Place spinach, Nama Shoyu, sesame oil, and garlic into a mixing bowl. Use your hands (you can wear gloves if you prefer) to mix well. Set aside for 20 minutes to allow spinach to wilt, soften, and marinate. Add scallion and sesame seeds.

To serve, transfer into serving bowl.

Will keep in fridge for 2 days.

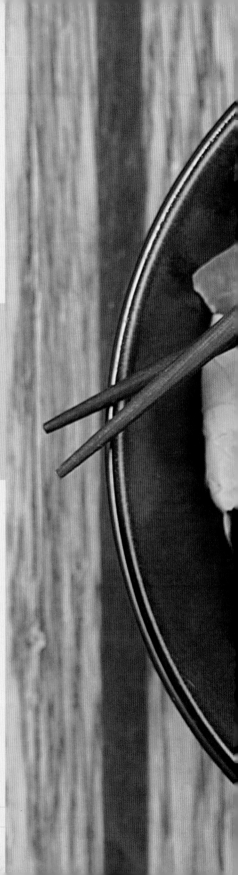

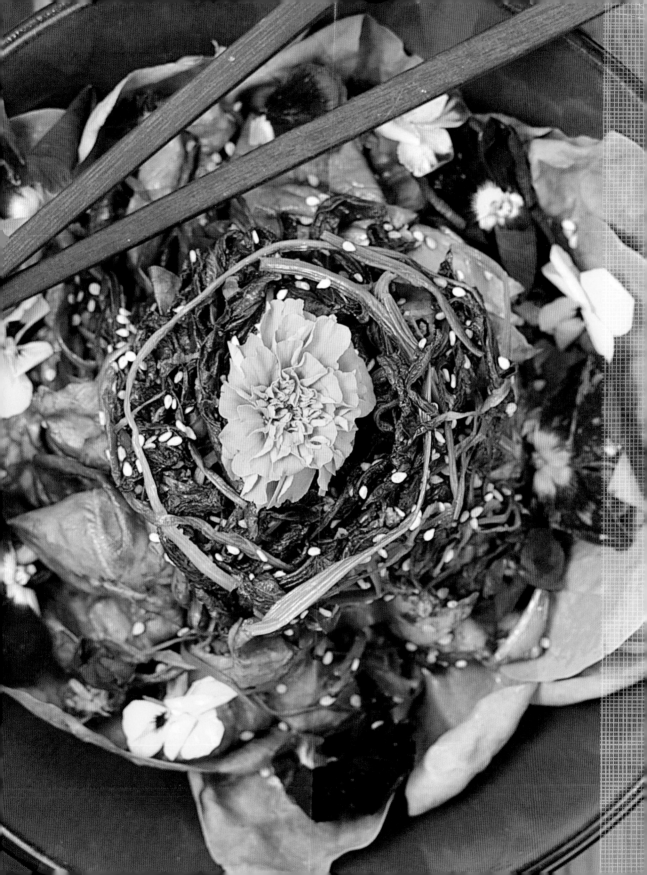

MEDICINAL MUSHROOMS

Mushrooms provide protein, fiber, B and C vitamins, calcium, potassium, and other minerals. Shiitake, along with maitake and reishi mushrooms, have been used for thousands of years in Asia for their phenomenal healing properties. They boost heart health; lower the risk of cancer; promote immune function; fight viruses, bacteria, and fungus; decrease inflammation; combat allergies; balance blood-sugar levels; and help our bodies detoxify. Lentinan in shiitake mushrooms stimulates the immune system, helps fight infection, and demonstrates antitumor activity.

Shiitake mushrooms are used to treat nutritional deficiencies and liver issues, maitake helps with the stomach and intestines, and reishi supports respiratory health.

Mushrooms are high in selenium, an antioxidant that works with vitamin E to protect our cells from age-accelerating free radical damage. Studies have shown male health professionals who consumed twice the recommend daily intake of selenium decreased their risk of prostate cancer by 65 percent. Most mushrooms have antitumor properties, and wood ear mushrooms help thin the blood to prevent clotting that contributes to heart disease.

Mushroom protein is a superior source compared to other vegetables due to its essential amino acid content, and 70 to 90 percent of the vegetable protein is easily digested.

When buying mushrooms, handle as little as possible. Never wash before storing. Remove from plastic container or bag and transfer into paper bag and store in fridge. Mushrooms last a few days in fridge, but are always best enjoyed immediately.

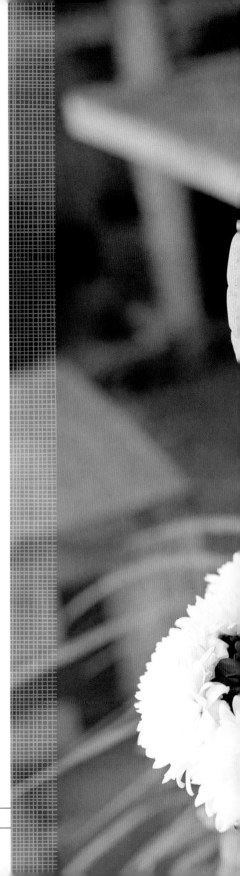

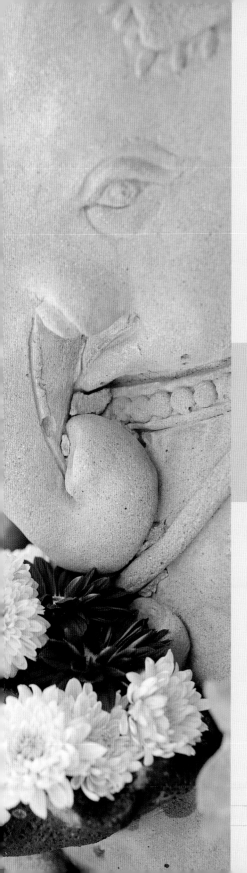

SHIITAKE MUSHROOM NAMUL

Korea

SERVES 4 AS SIDE DISH

In Asian and Buddhist cuisine, mushrooms of all varieties add the "meat" component to any meal or snack. Mushrooms are medicinal and used to boost our immune system and are a source of protein. You can use fresh or dried mushrooms. If you use dried, soak in double the amount of water and set aside to fully soften for several hours. About 1½ cups of dry will become about 2 cups once rehydrated.

2 cups cleaned and thinly sliced shiitake mushrooms

2 teaspoons toasted sesame oil

2 teaspoons Nama Shoyu

¼ teaspoon minced garlic

1 tablespoon sliced scallion

Pinch black pepper, to taste

Place mushrooms, sesame oil, Nama Shoyu, and garlic into a mixing bowl. Use your hands (you can wear gloves if you prefer) to mix well. Set aside 20 minutes or longer to soften and marinate. Add scallion and pepper and toss.

To serve, transfer to serving bowl.

Will keep for 2 days in fridge.

CRUSHED MIXED NORI

Korea

MAKES ¼ CUP

This dish is called *Kim Moo Chim* in Korean. *Kim* is Korean for nori and the word *moo chim* means to massage and mix by hand. Fast to make and a great add-on to any dish as a mineral-rich topping or side condiment.

Nori, 5 sheets, crushed or ground into flakes

½ red jalapeño, sliced thin

½ green jalapeño, sliced thin

2 tablespoons Nama Shoyu or tamari

1 tablespoon agave or brown rice syrup

1 tablespoon toasted sesame oil

1 tablespoon crushed sesame seeds

Place all ingredients into a bowl. Use your hands (you can wear gloves if you prefer) to massage and mix well. Serve immediately.

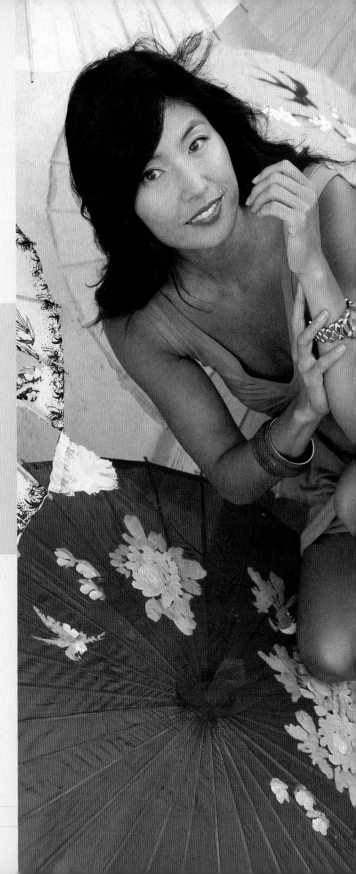

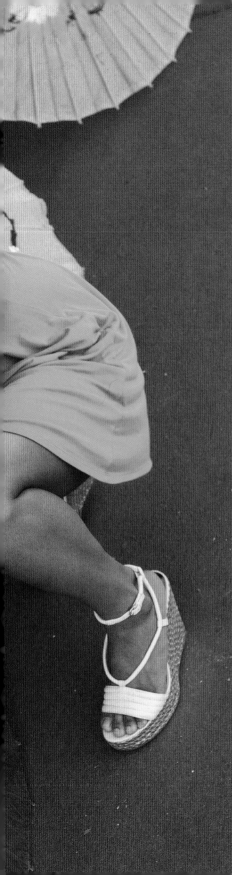

CHICORY AND ENDIVE NAMUL

Korea

SERVES 4 AS SIDE DISH

This is a modern-day namul that's gaining popularity in Korean communities in New York City. It's made with chicory leaves, also known as curly endive, and regular red and white endives. Chicory is crunchier and heartier than leaf lettuce and has a slightly bitter taste.

This namul has a sour and sweet flavor, as well as a slight bitter taste from the leaves.

2 cups thinly sliced chicory leaves

1 cup thinly sliced endives

1 tablespoon fresh lemon juice

1 tablespoon Nama Shoyu

1 teaspoon agave syrup

½ teaspoon minced garlic

¼ teaspoon red chile flakes, to taste

1 teaspoon sesame seeds

1 teaspoon chopped scallion

Place chicory, endives, lemon, Nama Shoyu, agave syrup, garlic, and chile into a bowl. Use your hands (you can wear gloves if you prefer) to mix well. Set aside for 30 to 40 minutes to marinate and soften. Add sesame seeds and scallion.

To serve, transfer to serving bowl.

Will keep for 2 days in fridge.

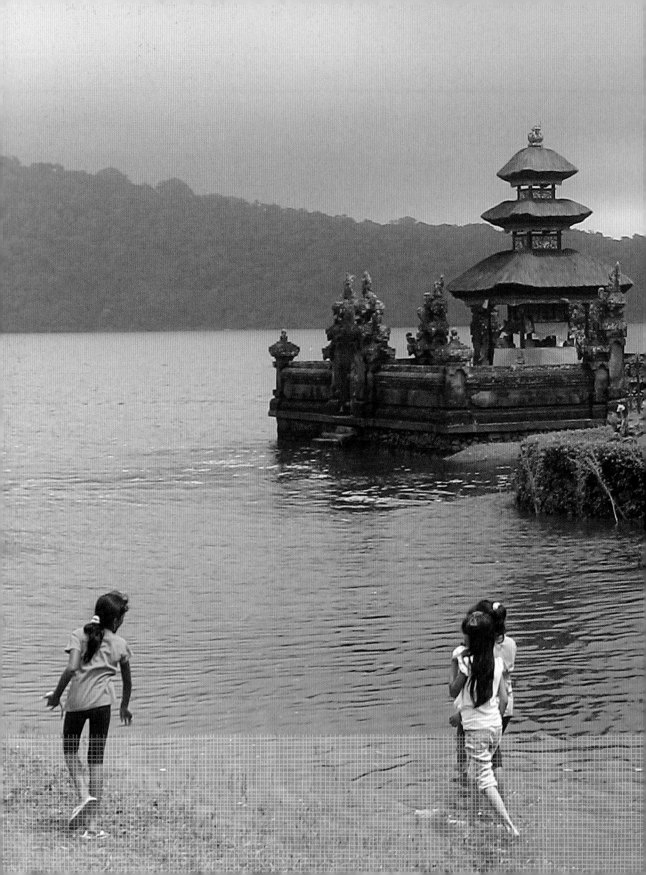

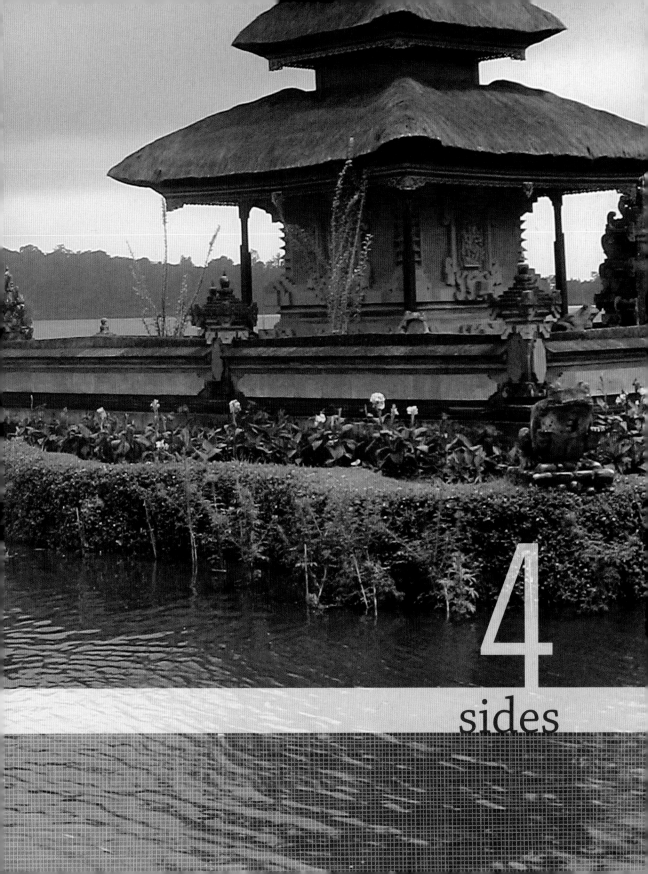

4
sides

NONTOXIC CLEANING RECIPES

I learned from my mom how to cut up an old t-shirt to use as a rag for cleaning, and I realize now how eco green our home was growing up. Dad always taught me to use less and to never waste. Today, that's called reduce, reuse, and recycle. And we never had toxic chemicals in our home.

As a general cleanser, I like to mix up Dr. Bronner's liquid soap with water in a spray bottle. Here're more recipes for making your own polish, deodorizer, and whitening powder.

FURNITURE POLISH

1 teaspoon lemon juice
1 pint of olive oil

Mix lemon and oil together and then apply a small amount to a clean cotton cloth and wipe wooden parts of furniture.

RUG DEODORIZER

Baking soda

Sprinkle baking soda on your rug. Wait 15 minutes or more before vacuuming.

MOTH REPELLENT

Cedar chips or
A sachet with dry lavender flowers, rosemary, or mint

WHITENING SCOURING POWDER

1 cup baking soda
2 teaspoons cream of tartar
⅛ cup borax
¼ cup grated lemon or orange peel

Mix well. Scrub using a damp sponge.

GLASS CLEANER

1½ cups vinegar
½ cup water

Combine in a spray bottle. Spray and wipe with a dry cloth.

A Clean Environment

Cleaning products were responsible for 10 percent of all toxic exposures reported to U.S. Poison Control centers in 2000. According to the U.S. Environmental Protection Agency (EPA), the air inside our home is two to ten times more hazardous than outside air, and is the #1 environmental health problem. Sometimes, air is a hundred times more contaminated indoors due to household cleaners and pesticides. These toxins are poisonous to our environment and human health.

You can always smell cleaning products, even when they are tightly sealed, because they outgas through plastic bottles and into the environment. Imagine what happens when these toxic poisons are sitting in a cabinet or under a sink at home. Cancer seldom comes from one exposure, but rather is the result of accumulation after prolonged low-level exposure to poisons.

In Canada, respiratory illness is the leading cause of hospitalization for children. And childhood asthma has increased exponentially. *Scientific American* reports that a baby crawling on the floor inhales the equivalent of four cigarettes a day due to the out-gassing of carpets, molds, mildews, fungi, and dust mites. After injuries, cancer is the leading cause of death in children five to nine years old.

Protect your body from accumulating toxins by seeking out healthy cleaning products and also avoiding unhealthy ones like these:

CORROSIVES

Found in most drain, oven, and toilet cleaners, corrosives contain the most dangerous chemicals including lye, hydrochloric acid, phosphoric acid, and sulfuric acid. Corrosives burn the skin and can explode.

AMMONIA

An eye and lung irritant that should be avoided by anyone with asthma or lung sensitivities. Dimethyl benzyl ammonia chloride is a pesticide ingredient in products that should be avoided.

BLEACH

Whiter whites aren't worth inhaling this irritant that gives off toxic fumes.

PHOSPHATES

Found in automatic dishwashing detergents as a water softener. They cause algae blooms in lakes and ponds and kill aquatic life when they run back into the environment. Phosphates were used in laundry products decades ago, but manufacturer have since reduced or eliminated phosphates. Phosphates are still found in dishwasher detergents, which contain about 30 to 40 percent phosphates.

PETROLEUM

Many cleaners are derived from petroleum and linked to health issues and damage mucous membranes. They wreak havoc on our environment, too. Avoid diethylene glycol, nonylphenol ethoxylate, and butyl cellosolve (found in many basic household cleaners such as window and floor cleaners). Butyl cellosolve is known to damage bone marrow, the nervous system, kidneys, and the liver.

ETHANOL

Also found in many common cleaning products, it is an eye and mucous membrane irritant and causes nervous system depression if inhaled or ingested.

When buying new cleaning products, make sure they don't contain surfactants, chlorine, or phosphates. Look for the labels "nontoxic" and "biodegradable." Or, better yet, just make your own cleansers.

Vegetables

Just as it is important to eliminate toxic cleaning products from our home and work environments, it's important to avoid eating poisonous chemicals in our food. In addition to fueling us up with super nutrients to combat aging and illness, enjoying fresh, whole organics means avoiding toxic pesticides, herbicides, artificial colors and flavors, and preservatives. Choose organic. In turn, this helps decrease overall stress, increasing our vitality and longevity.

Sides

 For times when you are craving something a bit warmer, all the recipes in this chapter can be heated up in a skillet or oven. I always recommend low heat. And, if you don't have a dehydrator yet, you can use your oven set on the lowest heat. To keep it more raw, prop the door open with a spoon handle. It's hardly eco to dehydrate this way, but hopefully it will inspire you to invest in a dehydrator. They are fun to have, and make crunchy, crispy textures that come only from drying.

KREAMED CURRY SAAG SPINACH

India

MAKES 4 SERVINGS

Saag Paneer is a popular Indian dish made by first pureeing and then cooking spinach with ghee or butter, ginger, onion, and curry spices. The spinach is then cooked with a homemade cheese (paneer). My simplified raw vegan version is made by first blending a cashew kream with cumin and coriander, then adding wilted spinach. My Cashew Kream has a flavor similar to paneer.

VEGETABLES

6 cups spinach

1 tablespoon finely chopped yellow onion

1 teaspoon finely chopped ginger

2 tablespoons liquid coconut oil,
    or extra-virgin olive oil

GARNISH (OPTIONAL)

2 tablespoons cilantro leaves

CASHEW KREAM (MAKES 2 CUPS)

1 teaspoon minced garlic

1 teaspoon sea salt

¼ teaspoon ground cumin

¼ teaspoon ground coriander

2 cups cashews

6 tablespoons fresh lemon juice

¼ cup filtered water

Place spinach, onion, ginger, and oil in mixing bowl, and toss to mix well. Set aside to soften.

To make Cashew Kream, place garlic, salt, cumin, coriander, and cashews into food processor. Process into powder. Add lemon juice and water and process to mix into a thick cream. Add spinach, and pulse gently to mix.

To serve, transfer into a serving bowl. Garnish with fresh cilantro leaves.

SERVING SUGGESTION: *Serve with 1 batch Dosa, page 177*

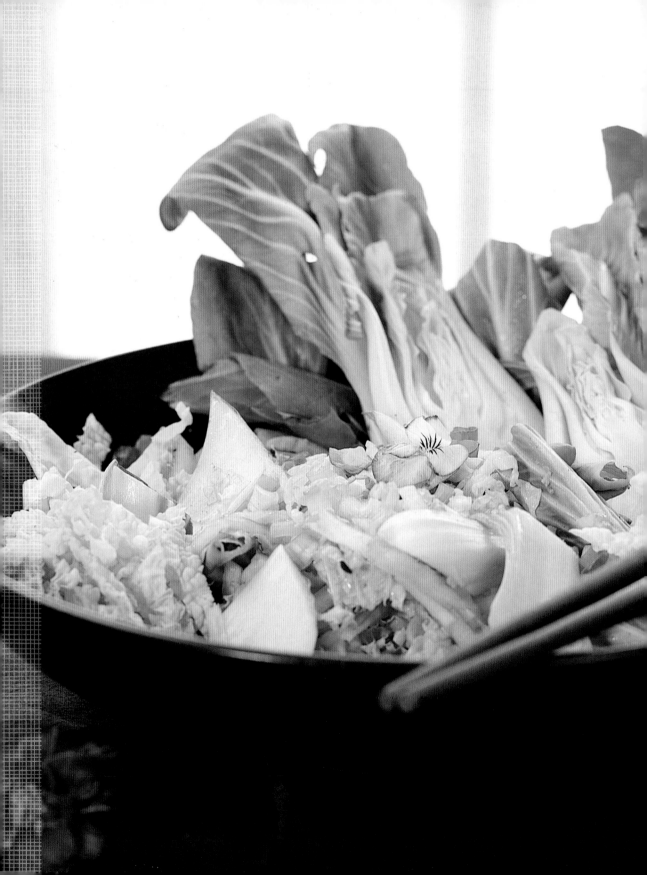

BABY BOK CHOY WITH CHINESE CABBAGE IN GINGER SAUCE

China

MAKES 4 SERVINGS

Napa cabbage comes from the Beijing region of China, is often used in East Asian cuisine, and is also called Chinese cabbage. In Korea, the leaves are used to make kimchi and wraps dipped in the Korean pepper sauce called *Gochujang* (see page 225).

Bok choy is another type of Chinese cabbage with dark green leaves, a sweet taste, and a crisp texture. Hong Kong supposedly has over twenty varieties of bok choy. We like to think "bigger is better" in the West, but the smaller version known as Shanghai or baby bok choy is desired for its tenderness in the East.

If you don't have baby bok choy available, you can use the larger bok choy variety instead.

2 cups sliced baby bok choy (trim ends and cut diagonally into 1½-inch strips)

1 cup thinly sliced napa cabbage

GINGER SAUCE

3 tablespoons Nama Shoyu

2 tablespoons apple cider vinegar

2 tablespoons agave syrup

1½ teaspoons grated ginger

GARNISH

1 tablespoon chopped scallion

Place sliced bok choy and napa cabbage into mixing bowl. Set aside.

To make sauce, whisk together Nama Shoyu, vinegar, agave syrup, and ginger in small bowl. Pour over bok choy and cabbage and toss to mix well. Set aside for at least 15 to 30 minutes to soften and marinate.

To serve, transfer into a serving dish. Garnish with scallion.

Will keep for 1 day in fridge.

BENEFITS OF GINGER

Ginger has been used as a natural remedy for ailments for centuries in both Chinese and Ayurvedic medicine and works wonders in the treatment of morning sickness, motion sickness, and nausea. It reduces pain and inflammation, is a natural heartburn remedy, and stimulates digestion. Ginger has been long used as a natural treatment for colds and flu and also provides migraine and menstrual pain relief. It's also a mood enhancer and contributes to stress relief. Ginger even kills cancer cells. University of Michigan Comprehensive Cancer Center found ovarian cancer cells die when ginger powder is applied directly to them.

Here're a few remedies:

MOTION SICKNESS

Take ¼ teaspoon fresh ginger 20 minutes before a car or boat trip for 4 hours of relief.

MIGRAINE

Take ⅓ teaspoon of fresh ginger when you feel a migraine coming on to stop pain before it starts.

ARTHRITIS PAIN

Take ½ teaspoon fresh ginger for arthritis relief.

MOUTH FRESHENER

Chew on a piece of ginger to clean and freshen your mouth.

Add more ginger into your diet by sprinkling grated ginger over rice, vegetables, soups. Adding ginger, sesame seeds, and nori strips spruces up any dish while also adding healthful nutrients. Or try this Ginger Lemonade recipe:

GINGER LEMONADE

MAKES 1 SERVING

1 tablespoon grated ginger
2 tablespoons lemon juice
1 to 2 tablespoons agave, maple syrup, or honey
1 cup filtered water

Combine all ingredients and serve over ice or at room temperature.

MAKE YOUR OWN ALMOND BUTTER

Making your own almond butter is simple, it just takes time. All you need is your food processor and about 15 minutes. It's always fresher to make your own anything, and helps to tread lighter on the planet, too, by using fewer resources like labels, packaging, manufacturing, and distributing.

In an ideal world, you always want to soak your nut and seeds before using. If soaking almonds first to make your butter, soak in filtered water about 8 hours, then discard soak water and rinse well. If you want, you can pop almonds out of their skin at this point by pinching between your thumb and first finger for a lighter colored butter. I don't bother peeling the skin off.

Make sure to dry soaked almonds completely before using by placing in your dehydrator at 104 degrees for 8 to 12 hours, until fully dry. You can place them in the sun to dry during hot, dry, summer months.

To make your butter, place about 2 cups of either unsoaked or soaked and fully dried almonds in your food processor with the S blade. Grind into small pieces, and scrape down the sides. If using soaked almonds, add a tablespoon of the oil of your choice, like raw almond or extra-virgin olive oil. You won't need additional oil if using unsoaked almonds.

Keep processing for up to 8 or 10 minutes, and your almonds will eventually begin to form one large ball in the food processor. If using soaked almonds, add one more tablespoon of oil if needed. Add oil gradually 1 tablespoon at a time. Maximum needed will be about 2 tablespoons.

Continue to process until the ball breaks apart inside the processor, and all the oils have mixed together. It will take anywhere from 12 to 15 minutes before you have the texture of a store-bought jarred almond butter.

Will keep for several weeks in jar in fridge, and even longer if using unsoaked almonds.

Optional: Add ½ teaspoon sea salt, and for a slightly sweeter flavor, 1 tablespoon honey or maple syrup or rice syrup at the very end. Try adding a tablespoon or 2 of cacao powder or carob powder.

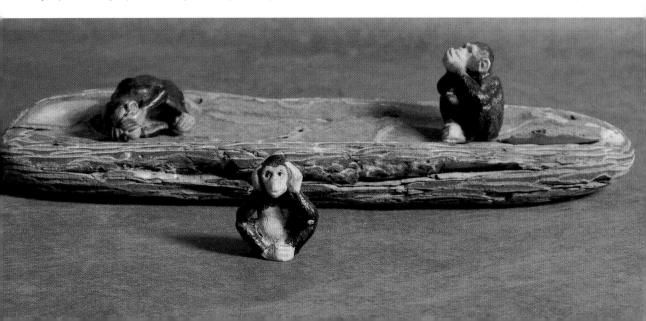

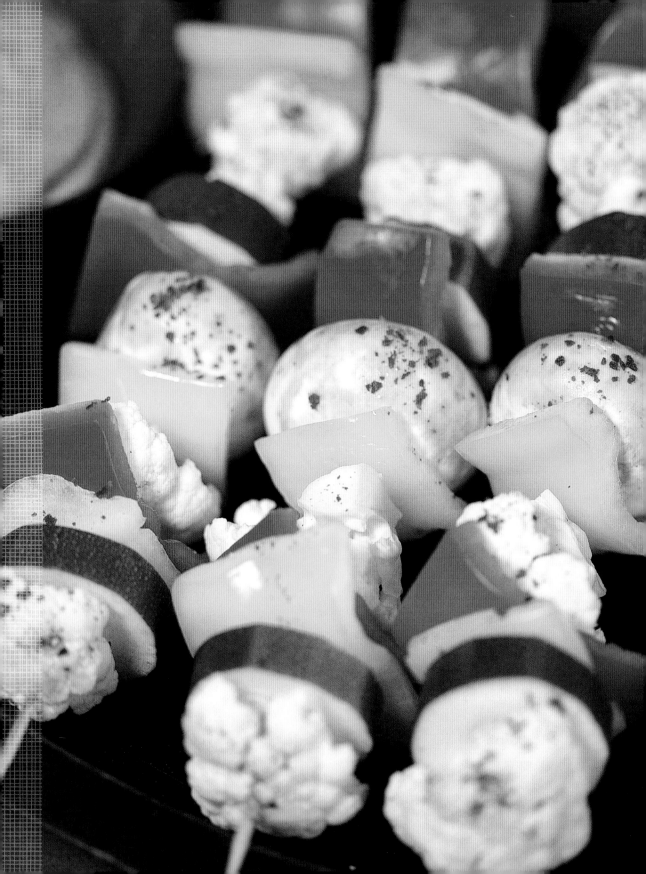

MIXED VEGETABLE SKEWERS WITH ALMOND BUTTER SAUCE

Hawaii

MAKES 4 SERVINGS

This recipe was inspired by my first trip to Hawaii last year, when I visited Oahu. Traditionally, skewers are marinated in a Teriyaki style sauce. In this recipe, I first marinate vegetables in my Sesame Romaine Salad Dressing. Then later I pair beautifully colored vegetables and sweet pineapple with a simple and delicious Almond Butter Sauce.

Feel free to mix up the vegetables to include whatever is in season, available, or your favorites.

SKEWERS
½ cup cubed red bell peppers (about ½ medium pepper)

½ cup bite-size pieces cauliflower florets

½ cup sliced green beans, cut diagonally into 1-inch pieces

½ cup cubed zucchini (about ½ medium zucchini)

½ cup cubed pineapple

½ cup whole white or cremini mushrooms

MARINADE
1 batch Sesame Romaine Salad Dressing, page 62

ALMOND BUTTER SAUCE (MAKES 1 CUP)
½ cup almond butter

⅓ cup fresh lemon juice

3 tablespoons liquid coconut oil (melt the solid coconut oil by placing the jar into a bowl of hot water)

3 tablespoons Bragg Liquid Aminos

GARNISH (OPTIONAL)
2 cups spinach

2 cups shredded green cabbage

1 cup mung bean sprouts

Place all skewer ingredients into a large mixing bowl. Toss with Sesame Romaine Salad Dressing. Set aside to marinate at least 20 to 30 minutes. Then, assemble by evenly distributing vegetables along wooden skewers.

To make your Almond Butter Sauce, place all ingredients into a blender and blend to mix well.

To serve, portion spinach, cabbage, and mung bean sprouts onto 4 serving dishes. Place skewers on top of your bed of greens. Serve with a side of Almond Butter Sauce.

Marinated skewers will keep for 2 days in fridge. Almond Butter Sauce will keep for 4 to 5 days in fridge when stored separately.

VEGETABLE TEMPURA WITH ORANGE LEMONGRASS DIPPING SAUCE

Japan

MAKES 4 SERVINGS

A creamy batter is used to coat your favorite vegetables, which are then dehydrated to make a delicious breaded tempura crust, without frying. I like to mix cashews with pumpkin seeds. Feel free to mix, or just use one or the other. If you don't have a dehydrator yet, you can make this recipe in your oven on the lowest setting. Propping the door open will keep the temperature lower but is hardly eco. Hopefully, you'll be inspired to add a dehydrator to your kitchen.

Serve with a fragrant lemongrass dipping sauce.

TEMPURA BATTER

1 cup peeled and chopped zucchini
    (about 1 medium zucchini)

1 cup cashews and/or pumpkin seeds

2 tablespoons nutritional yeast

1 tablespoon extra-virgin olive oil

½ teaspoon sea salt

⅓ cup water, as needed

VEGETABLES

A total of 5 cups of your favorites like:

Broccoli, broken into tiny bite-size pieces

Onion, thinly sliced

Carrot, thinly sliced

String bean, cut into 2-inch lengths

Bell pepper, red or green, sliced into spears

Asparagus, sliced diagonally into
    2-inch lengths

ORANGE LEMONGRASS DIPPING SAUCE

⅓ cup orange juice

2 tablespoons lemon zest

1 tablespoon finely chopped lemongrass

2 tablespoons Nama Shoyu or Bragg Liquid
    Aminos

1 teaspoon agave syrup

Place all batter ingredients into your blender with least amount of water as possible. Blend to mix into a smooth creamy consistency.

Put all vegetables into a mixing bowl. Toss and massage with batter to coat well. Place in single layer onto three dehydrator trays and dry at 104°F for 7 to 10 hours, to desired level of dryness. You want the batter to be crisp, and the vegetables to be softened.

To make dipping sauce, whisk together ingredients in small bowl.

To serve, transfer dipping sauce to serving bowl. Place on center of a large platter with tempura vegetables arranged around it.

Sauce will keep 3 days in fridge. Tempura is best enjoyed immediately, or store in airtight container in fridge, and dehydrate a couple of hours before serving again.

SERVING SUGGESTION: *serve on top of Jicama "Rice" with Sliced Scallions and Sesame Oil, page 222.*

WHAT IS NUTRITIONAL YEAST?

Nutritional yeast is yellow in color and comes in either a powder or flake form that's sprinkled over food to add nutrient value and flavor. Its nutty, "cheesy" taste makes it popular with vegans. It can be sprinkled over salads, soups, and gravies.

Nutritional yeast is grown on enriched purified cane and beet molasses and is a reliable food source for vitamin B-12. Find it in the bulk or supplement section of your natural food store.

MARINATED SHIITAKE MUSHROOM DUMPLINGS WITH LEMON SOY DIPPING SAUCE

Korea

MAKES 4 SERVINGS

Mushrooms are marinated in a raw soy sauce with toasted sesame oil and a pinch of chile pepper, then used to fill wrappers of thinly sliced, marinated daikon radish. Serve with a tart dipping sauce, all inspired by how it's done in Korea.

It works best to slice a daikon that's large in diameter into paper-thin circles to make folding into wrappers easier. Another option is to use two smaller or thicker circles to sandwich your filling instead.

Daikon is very low in calories with only 18 calories per ¼-cup serving and is a great food for weight loss. Daikon provides 34 percent of the RDA for vitamin C and contains active enzymes that aid digestion of fatty oils and starchy foods.

Select a daikon that feels heavy and has a lustrous skin and fresh leaves.

MUSHROOM FILLING

2 cups sliced shiitake mushrooms

1 tablespoon toasted sesame oil, or extra-virgin olive oil

2 teaspoons Nama Shoyu or Bragg Liquid Aminos

A pinch to ⅛ teaspoon Korean chile powder or cayenne, to taste

DUMPLING WRAPPERS

3- to 4-inch length of a fat daikon radish, sliced into about 1 cup of very thin rounds

2 teaspoons Nama Shoyu or Bragg Liquid Aminos

LEMON SOY DIPPING SAUCE (MAKES ½ CUP)

½ cup Nama Shoyu

3 tablespoons apple cider vinegar

2 tablespoons extra-virgin olive oil

1 teaspoon grated ginger

1 teaspoon lemon zest

Place all filling ingredients into a bowl and toss to mix well. Set aside to marinate and soften for at least 20 minutes.

Place wrapper ingredients into a mixing bowl. Toss to mix well. Set aside for 10 minutes to marinate and soften.

In a small mixing bowl, combine dipping sauce ingredients. Whisk to mix well.

Assemble by scooping about 1 teaspoon marinated mushrooms into center of marinated radish round. Fold into semi circle. Repeat.

To serve, transfer dumplings onto serving dishes and serve with dipping sauce.

Dumplings will keep 1 day in fridge, though best enjoyed immediately as they will release water. Dipping sauce will keep for 4 days in fridge.

SERVING SUGGESTION: *Dipping sauce makes for a great dressing on salads, too.*

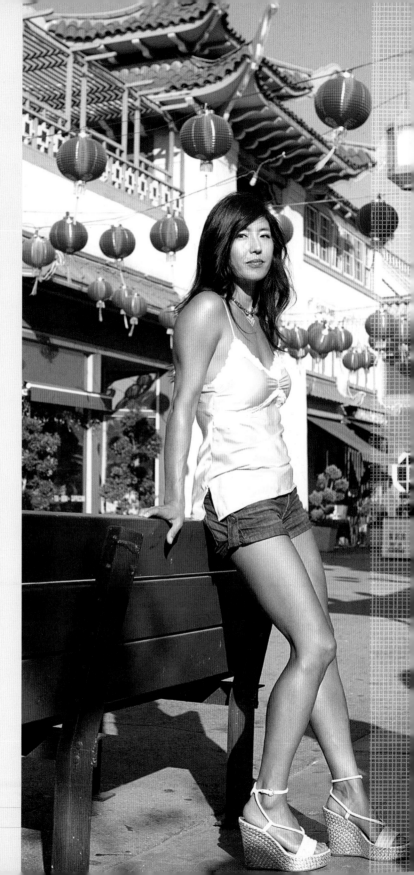

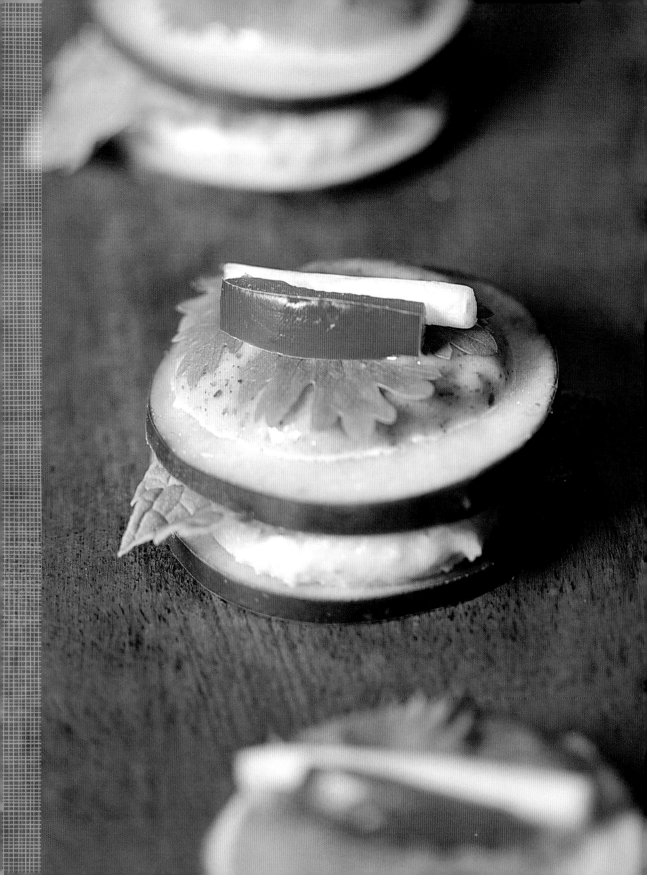

CILANTRO CHEEZE–STUFFED CUCUMBER RAVIOLI

Vietnam

MAKES 4 SERVINGS

Many cultures have a recipe for small packets of food. From mandu in Korea, to dumplings in China, to ravioli in Italy. This is my fusion of a Western-style raw food ravioli inspired by a deconstructed Vietnamese-style spring roll.

Zesty cheeze is sandwiched between slices of refreshing cucumber with fresh mint. Topped with a creamy Almond Butter Sauce, beautiful cilantro, and red chile pepper, it's full of flavor, with a colorful presentation.

CHEEZE

1 teaspoon minced garlic

1 teaspoon sea salt

2 cups cashews

½ cup fresh cilantro

6 tablespoons fresh lemon juice

¼ cup filtered water, as needed

RAVIOLI

1 cucumber, sliced into thin circles

¼ cup fresh mint leaves

GARNISH

½ batch Almond Butter Sauce, page 117

2 tablespoons cilantro leaves

2 tablespoons chopped mung bean sprouts, cut into 2-inch lengths

2 tablespoons sliced Thai chile pepper, Serrano, or other red pepper, seeded and sliced into 1-inch matchsticks

To make cheeze, place garlic, salt, and cashews into food processor. Process into powder. Add cilantro, lemon juice, and just enough water to make a thick consistency.

Assemble ravioli by sandwiching about a teaspoon of cheeze and one mint leaf between two cucumber circles.

Serve by transferring ravioli to serving dishes. Top with dollop of Almond Butter Sauce. Garnish by placing one cilantro leaf, one mung bean sprout, and one piece of Thai chile pepper on top of each ravioli. Enjoy immediately.

LOTUS ROOT CHIPS WITH PINE NUT MUSTARD SAUCE

Japan

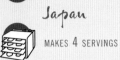

MAKES 4 SERVINGS

Lotus root is in the water lily family and grows in ponds in tropical areas throughout Asia. All of the plant is edible, and the root is most commonly eaten. It's off-white in color, similar to a parsnip, and grows up to 4 feet long and 2½ inches wide. The center of the root if filled with holes that keep the plant buoyant in water. These holes make a beautiful, symmetric pattern that looks like a snowflake when the root is sliced crosswise into rounds. You can find lotus root at Asian markets, usually year round.

Use a knife or peeler to remove the outer skin and put slices immediately into a lemon water bath to slow oxidation. Enjoy as is or marinate and eat slices as you would carrot sticks or celery with dips. These beautiful slices have a mild flavor and substantial crunch, making them easy to enjoy on their own and paired with dips and sauces.

You can also pop slices into your dehydrator for a few hours to soften, but not too long, as they become rock-hard when completely dry. (I messed up my first batch and gave the chips to Kanga, my pooch, who enjoyed chomping down on the hard bits!)

Store the whole root in your fridge for 2 to 3 weeks.

Lotus root is a symbol of purity and life, and is eaten for New Year's celebrations in China.

LEMON WATER BATH

4 cups water

2 tablespoons fresh lemon juice

CHIPS

4-inch piece of lotus root

1½ teaspoon Nama Shoyu

⅛ teaspoon cayenne powder

SAUCE

1 batch Pine Nut Mustard Sauce, page 125

PINE NUT MUSTARD SAUCE

Japan

MAKES 1 CUP

Begin by placing water and lemon juice into a mixing bowl.

Next, wash and peel your lotus root using a knife or peeler. Cut root crosswise into rounds that are about ⅛ inch thick. Place into bath immediately upon slicing to prevent oxidation. You will have about 2 cups of sliced lotus root.

Pat slices dry using a towel. Place into mixing bowl with Nama Shoyu and cayenne. Toss to mix and coat well. Enjoy immediately, or set aside for 30 minutes or longer to marinate and soften. Enjoy alone or with dipping sauce.

If dehydrating, spread in single layer onto one lined dehydrator tray. Dry at 104°F degrees for 2 to 3 hours, to desired texture. Avoid drying completely.

Serve with Pine Nut Mustard Sauce in a bowl as a dip.

SERVING SUGGESTION: *Lotus Root Chips make a beautiful garnish for any dish.*

According to Chinese Medicine, the spicy or pungent taste of mustard warms and works with the stomach and lung meridians. Mustard regulates Qi, clears dampness, expels phlegm, eases chest congestion, reduces swelling, and alleviates joint and body pain.

This recipe is for a pungent and sweet dipping sauce made with apple juice to counter the heat of hot mustard. Rich pine nuts add an aromatic tone. Use mustard powder or your favorite jarred mustard for this recipe. I prefer hot mustard like the Chinese style, but you can also use an English, Dijon, or Japanese yellow mustard (karashi).

To make a dressing out of this sauce, add some sesame or olive oil for a sweet and sour vinaigrette.

1 tablespoon Nama Shoyu

3 tablespoons apple cider vinegar

1 teaspoon mustard powder, or 2 tablespoons prepared mustard

2 tablespoons agave syrup or maple syrup

1 teaspoon sea salt

½ cup apple juice or filtered water

1 teaspoon ground flax meal

¼ cup finely chopped pine nuts

In mixing bowl or small jar, whisk or shake to mix together all ingredients.

Will keep for a week in fridge stored in airtight container.

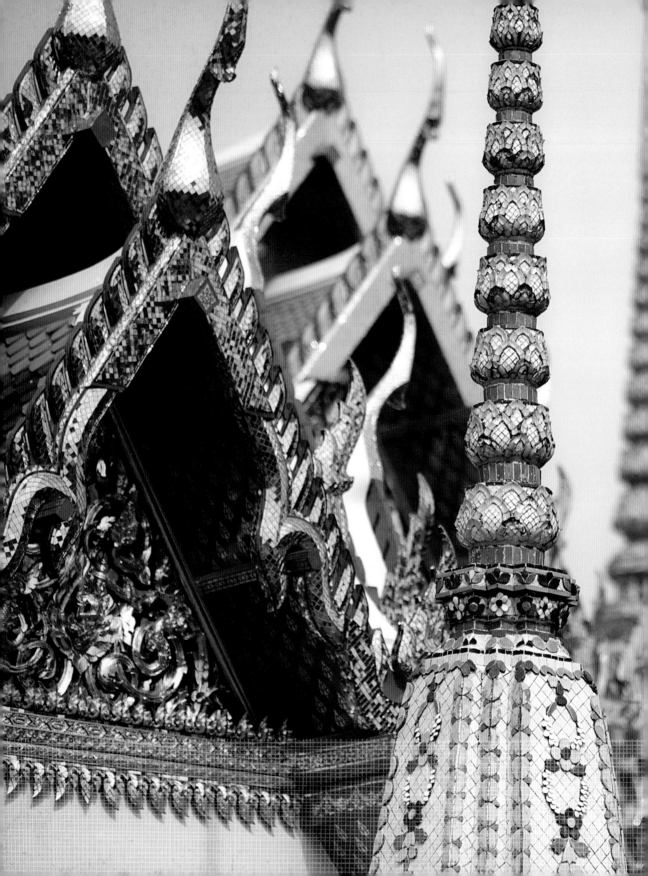

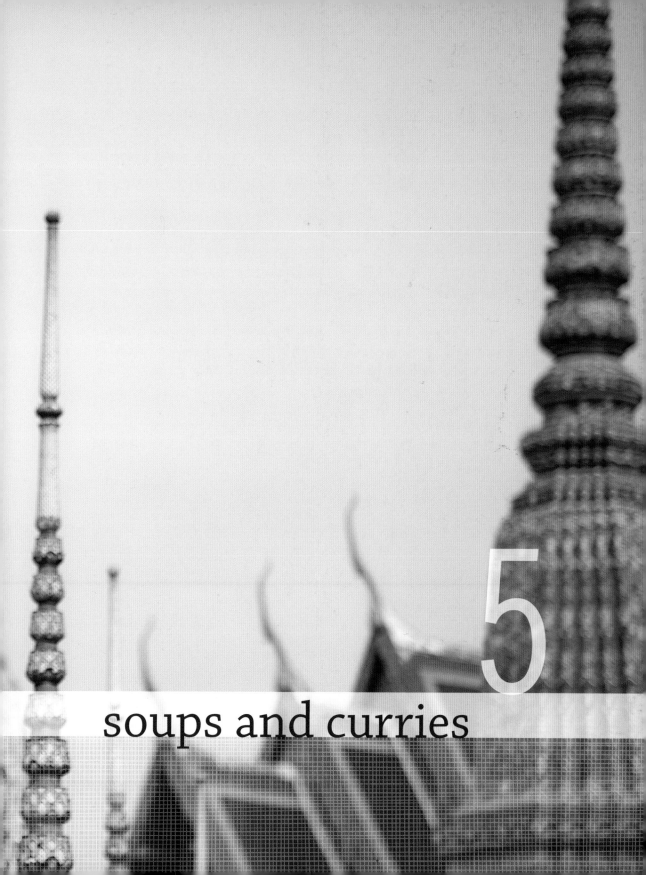

soups and curries

5

Toxin-Free Living

Toxins come at us through our environment, what we put into our bodies, and what we put onto our skin and hair. All these toxins build up in our body over time before showing up later as an illness and even cancer. Having negative thoughts also contributes to a toxic lifestyle.

BEAUTY

Our skin is our largest organ, so anything we put on our skin is absorbed into our bodies as if we'd eaten it. So, the same principle I apply to my food I apply to my beauty regimen. I try to avoid manufactured, processed products, and instead do my best to go straight to the source, Mother Nature.

Lemon juice is full of vitamin C found in many skin care products. Fresh lemon juice works great to lighten dark spots on skin. Organic ingredients like coconut or jojoba oil are great for skin and hair.

Asian natural care systems believe vitality and beauty come from within our body. In Asia, the belief is that beauty comes from proper nutrition that supports our inner functions in absorption, digestion, and elimination, toning up our inner system first, then working on our outer skin and hair.

Raw foods are nourishing, cleansing, detoxifying, and help build a clean, lean, strong, healthy body from the inside out. The healthier we are on the inside, the more it shows up on the outside as clear skin and shiny strong hair and nails that give us a beautiful glow.

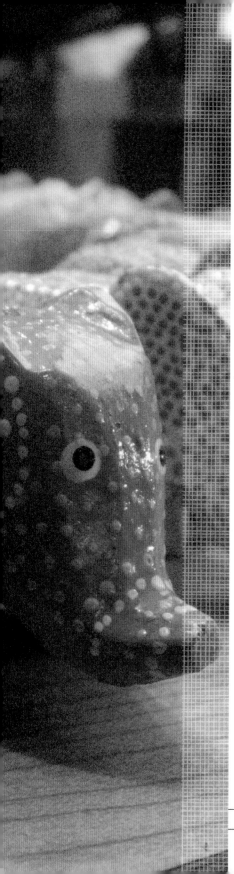

CHOOSE TOXIN-FREE PRODUCTS

Beauty and personal care products are loaded with harsh and harmful chemicals like triclosan (an antibacterial) and polyethylene. Both are associated with endocrine disruption, organ-system toxicity, and skin irritation.

Here are some ingredients to look out for and avoid:

SODIUM LAURYL SULPHATE

SLS is an irritant and is found in most shampoos, conditioners, body washes, and bubble baths. It's a detergent and foaming agent that irritates eyes, skin, and mucous membranes.

NANOPARTICLES

The latest new toxin used in a range of products including lipsticks to foundations. They enter the bloodstream to cause inflammation and irritation.

PARABENS

A toxic preservative found in cosmetics, toothpaste, and antibacterial agents. Parabens have been linked to cancer. The four main parabens are methyl, ethyl, propyl, and butyl parabens.

TITANIUM DIOXIDE

A suspected carcinogen used as a pigment and thickener for many cosmetic and skincare products. It's harmful to the environment, acidifies rivers and seas, and damages ecosystems in nature.

Many cosmetics contain unbelievable ingredients like formaldehyde, really! Visit http://safecosmetics.org/ for more info and to watch a great animation "The Story of Cosmetics."

>>>

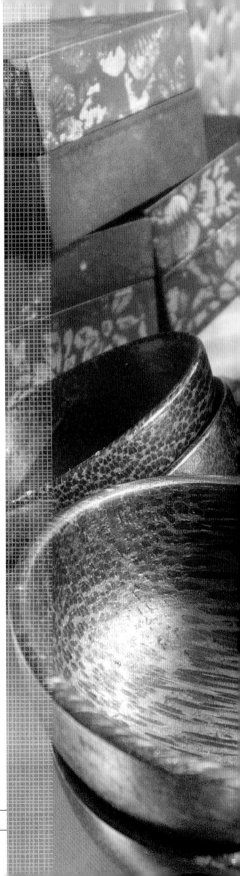

>>>

Other Keys for Toxin-Free Beauty

ORGANIC? CHECK THE LOGOS

Manufacturers aren't required to obtain organic certification when making organic claims. So, look for products that carry logos from the Soil Association, Ecocert, or USDA Organic (U.S. Department of Agriculture) to ensure they have been deemed safe for human health.

HAIR SPRAY

Consider skipping it if you can. Most contain phthalates known to disrupt our hormones and have been linked to numerous health scares including birth defects. If you need to spray, choose hairspray made with natural ingredients in a pump rather than an aerosol can.

NAIL POLISH

I choose buffed, naked, and natural nails. Nail varnish smells poisonous and is full of toxins like toluene, acetone, formaldehyde, phthalates, and colors that won't break down in nature. I feel like nail polish suffocates my nails and keeps them from breathing.

If you're hooked on pretty-colored nails, do seek out the BDIH label. It's a German certification guaranteeing eco and natural plant oils and herbal and floral extracts from managed cultivation. BDIH-certified products do not include organic synthetic dyes, synthetic fragrances, or mineral oil derivatives.

>>>

>>>

SUN DAMAGE

My tune has changed since my first book, when I didn't wear sunblock. Now that I'm older, I can see aging in my skin and spots from the sun. So for vanity reasons, I do wear a layer of sunblock when going outside in the middle of the day and wash it off when I come back inside. I practice moderation, and though sun block is not natural or 100 percent clean, I wear it only occasionally for an hour or two. I always wear a hat and sunglasses as well.

Skin cancer rates continue to rise, and one theory is that the increase is due to chemicals in sunblock itself. So avoid parabens, PABAs (para-aminobenzoic acid), padimate-O, parsol 1289, benzephenone, homosalate, and octy-methoxycinnamate (octinoxate).

When shopping for sunblock, always choose natural brands, or better yet, make your own moisturizing sunblock and sunscreen to nourish and prevent damage from harmful rays. Here're three homemade recipes for avoiding scary ingredients that are bad for your skin and your health.

SOOTHING

Coconut oil and olive oil block and reduce about 20 percent of the sun's burning rays, while aloe soothes and moisturizes.

1 tablespoon aloe vera juice
1 tablespoon coconut oil or extra-virgin olive oil

Mix and apply to exposed skin hourly.

HELICHRYSUM SUNBLOCK

Helichrysum is an essential oil effective as a natural sunblock.

1 drop helichrysum oil, an essential oil,
    very potent, use sparingly
25 drops coconut or extra-virgin olive oil

Mix and apply to exposed skin every few hours.

HELICHRYSUM SESAME SUNBLOCK

Sesame oil blocks or reduces about 30 percent of the sun's burning rays, and mixed with helichrysum, aloe, and chamomile makes a moisturizing, soothing sunblock.

2 tablespoons sesame oil
½ tablespoon aloe vera juice
3 drops helichrysum oil
2 drops chamomile oil

Mix and apply to exposed skin every hour.

POSITIVE THOUGHTS

Beyond decreasing or eliminating toxic chemicals in and around us, shedding toxic thoughts in our mind is just as important for helping to live a Super Life, longer. To live longer feeling deprived and filled with negative thoughts, resentment, or unhappiness sounds like torture to me. Instead, I strive to live a long Super Life filled with positive thoughts, compassionate people, good friends, family, laughter, healthy clean food and water, exercise and fitness, meditation, yoga, sunshine, and love.

I have my good and bad days like anyone. On bad days, my gratitude practice helps me get back on track. I'll list out my blessings including waking up here in America, having running water, flushing toilets, my health, my eyesight, my family and friends, Kanga my dog, and the knowledge of and access to healthy food and clean water. The list goes on and on and on.

It also helps to focus my attention on what I want, rather than worrying about what I don't want to happen, or what other people do, say, or think. Forgiveness and letting go is hard for me, but I do continue to practice it. Giving back is a big one. It helps me feel connected when I volunteer with a local community gardening organization teaching underprivileged children how to garden and make food, and when I help provide meals to cancer and HIV/AIDS patients in LA. And, by simply sitting in the sun or going on a walk in the woods, I connect back with nature. Before I know it, I'm feeling happy again.

>>>

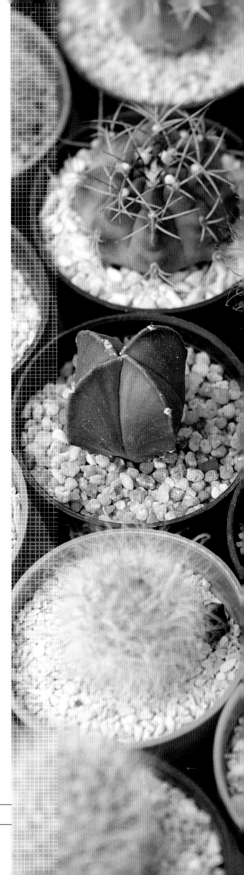

>>>

DAILY HAPPINESS TIPS

These are some of the things I strive to practice each day. I call it "practice" because it takes work, but over time, becomes easier to do.

Forgive

No one is perfect, and mistakes are only mistakes when they aren't given a chance to be corrected. Remember to also forgive ourselves.

Compassion

Treat others as you want to be treated, with love, patience, tolerance, humility, and forgiveness.

Make Amends

The only person who suffers when we hold on to resentment and bitterness is us.

Be Generous

With your time, energy, and resources. I would not be where I am today if it weren't for all the people who took time to help me when I needed it. Making time to help someone else is really rewarding.

Be Kind

Mom always taught me to be kind, including to those I know and those I don't know yet.

Inner Happiness

Try not to be affected by what goes on around you, focus within yourself, do good around you, and create your own happy reality.

Make a Difference

Give back and make a difference in your own neighborhood and community without seeking money or financial gain.

Faith, Hope, and Inspiration

Find something to believe in, whether it's that all people are inherently good, the god that's within each and every one of us, or Gaia and Mother Earth.

Soups

Soups are made by whisking or blending together ingredients to make a base, and for most, vegetables are added on before serving as toppings.

Soups can be a meal all on their own or an appetizer or a side dish. They travel well and are a good option for taking with you on the road and for lunch at the office.

 If you're craving a warm or hot soup or curry, any of these recipes (except the first) can be heated up in a saucepan to your desired temperature. I like to check temperature using my finger. When it's warm to the touch, it's hot enough for me. I prefer keeping my temperatures below 104°F for maximum nutritional and enzyme benefits.

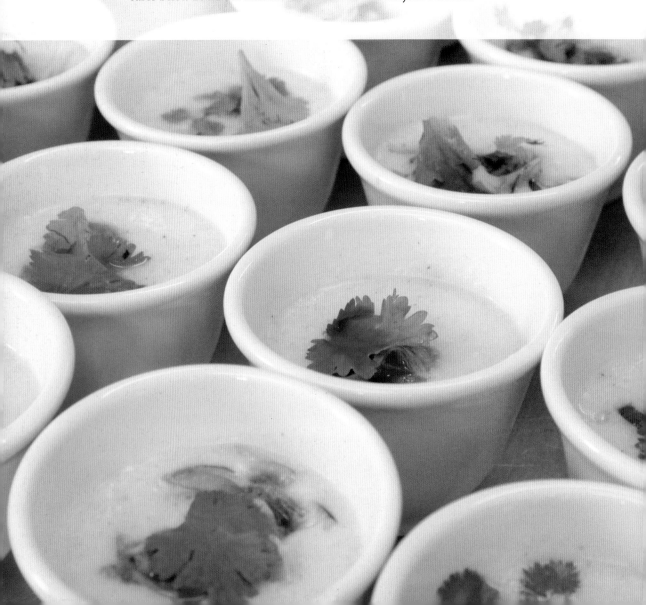

CHILLED CUCUMBER SOUP

Korea

MAKES 4 SERVINGS

A very simple sweet and sour soup that's like a floating cucumber salad with a tartness that stimulates the appetite. This refreshing soup is great on a hot summer day. Serve this cooling soup as a side with any spicy meal.

VEGETABLES

4 mini cucumbers, or ½ English cucumber, sliced into matchsticks, about 2 cups

2 shallots, cut into matchsticks, about ½ cup

1 teaspoon fine sea salt

BROTH

¼ cup rehydrated wakame

1 teaspoon minced garlic

Pinch chile powder

3 tablespoons apple cider vinegar

4 tablespoons agave syrup or brown rice syrup

1 tablespoon Nama Shoyu or tamari

3 cups filtered water

GARNISH

1 teaspoon seeded and sliced hot cherry pepper or red chile, cut into thin rings, to taste

1 teaspoon sesame seeds

1 cup ice cubes

Place cucumbers, shallots, and salt into a large mixing bowl. Toss to mix well. Set aside to soften for about 10 minutes.

Next, add all the broth ingredients except the water to cucumbers. Massage to mix well with your hands. Add water, mix, and then place in refrigerator to chill.

To serve, scoop into four serving bowls, and garnish with red pepper, sesame seeds, and ice. Enjoy immediately.

MISO SOUP WITH SPINACH AND BEAN SPROUTS

Korea

MAKES 4 SERVINGS

Miso is a living food. It starts off cooked, but it's then fermented and contains living enzymes. The best way to enjoy miso is raw, and even in Asia, miso is added to warm, never boiling, water so as to not damage the enzymes and beneficial probiotic bacteria. Pasteurization kills beneficial bacteria, so make sure to use an unpasteurized miso. See Miso sidebar, page 64.

Most natural food stores have mung bean sprouts, but if you can't find any, just use another sprout like alfalfa.

VEGETABLES

1 cup mung bean sprouts

2 cups washed, coarsely chopped spinach

2 tablespoons extra-virgin olive oil

BROTH

3 tablespoons miso, unpasteurized, any color

3 cups water

2 tablespoons extra-virgin olive oil

1 teaspoon minced garlic

GARNISH

2 tablespoons diced scallion

Marinate sprouts and spinach by tossing with extra-virgin olive oil. Set aside to soften.

To make your broth, whisk together miso and a small amount of water. Slowly add remaining water, oil, and garlic. You can also blend if you want instead.

To serve, transfer broth into four serving bowls. Top with marinated sprouts and spinach and garnish with scallion. Enjoy immediately.

Broth will keep for 4 to 5 days when stored separately in fridge.

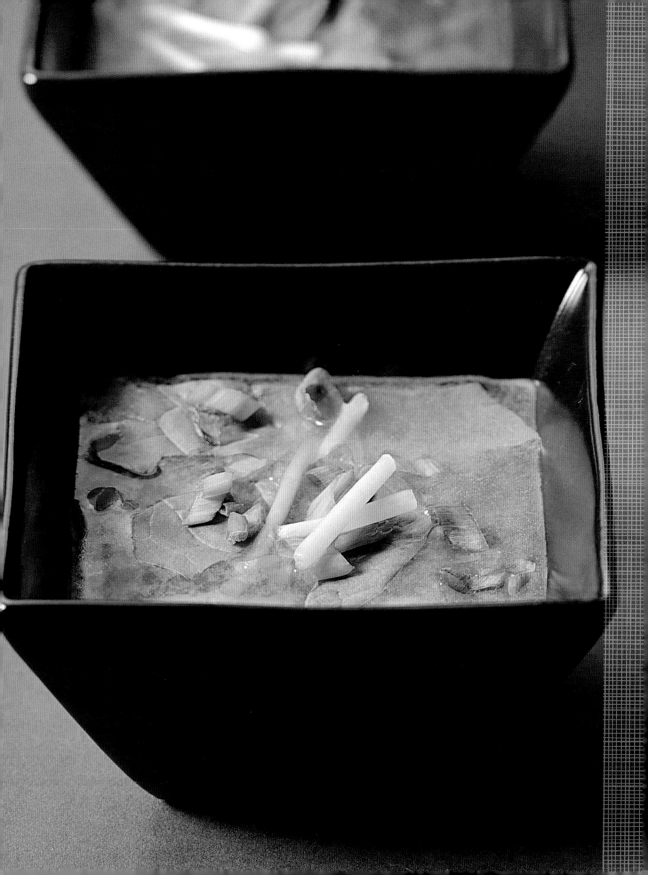

SESAME MUSHROOM SOUP

Korea

MAKES 4 SERVINGS

A simple and quick soup made by blending together tahini with water to make a creamy base topped with a marinated mushroom mix of shiitake, white, and enoki mushrooms. Feel free to substitute with your favorite or available mushrooms. Garnish with sesame seeds. Provides a great dose of calcium for building strong bones and teeth, plus a blast of vitamin E for beautifying and slowing down the signs of aging.

MARINATED MUSHROOMS
4 shiitake mushrooms, cut into matchstick strips

6 white mushrooms, cut into ¼-inch slices

1 bunch enoki mushrooms, split into separate bunches

¼ cup Nama Shoyu

2 tablespoons toasted sesame oil

SOUP
3 cups filtered water

½ cup tahini

2 tablespoons agave syrup

GARNISH
2 tablespoons crushed sesame seeds

Marinate mushrooms by placing all ingredients into a mixing bowl, toss well. Set aside to soften for at least 20 minutes.

Blend soup ingredients.

To serve, transfer soup base to four serving bowls. Top with marinated mushrooms and the marinade. Garnish with sesame seeds, and enjoy immediately.

SEAWEED SOUP WITH SHIITAKE AND DAIKON

Japan

MAKES 4 SERVINGS

An easy, delicious clear broth made with just three vegetables. Great on its own and also as a base for other soups. The flavors are of soy, mushrooms, and onion, and the combination of seaweed, daikon, and shiitake gives this broth its medicinal value (see sidebars on Medicinal Mushrooms, page 102, and Ancient Longevity Secret: Seaweed, page 140).

TOPPING
2 cups sliced shiitake mushrooms
¼ cup thinly sliced yellow onion
1 cup diced daikon radish
½ cup Nama Shoyu

SOUP
5 cups filtered water
½ cup dried wakame and/or dulse
2 tablespoons agave syrup

GARNISH
Ground black pepper, to taste

Place all topping ingredients into mixing bowl. Toss to mix well. Set aside to marinate and soften for 20 minutes or longer.

To make soup, place all the soup ingredients into a large mixing bowl. Set aside for 20 minutes or longer, until dried seaweed is hydrated. Using warmer water will shorten soak time.

To serve, transfer soup to serving bowls. Top with the shiitake mixture and garnish with black pepper.

Will keep for 1 day in fridge.

ANCIENT LONGEVITY SECRET: SEAWEED

Seaweed, a sea vegetable and marine algae that photosynthesizes like plants do on land, is an ancient Asian health secret. It's a true super food perfect for fueling a Super Life!

Seaweeds convert rich minerals in the ocean into an edible form. Rich in iodine, many Asian cultures ingested them as the main source for preventing goiter and treating thyroid conditions. They are a great source of iron, magnesium, and folate (vitamin B-9), calcium, sodium, potassium, iodine, zinc, and other vitamins, minerals, and trace elements.

Though part of the plant kingdom, sea vegetables are a complete protein source. They're one of the richest sources of protein in nature, up to 38 percent, and high in vitamin B-12.

Kelp, a sea vegetable, has been documented as being used for its iodine to treat obesity since as early as 1862. Iodine works with the thyroid to balance our metabolism. Seaweeds are low in calories, fat, and carbohydrates, making them a great weight loss food.

Seaweed has been shown to cleanse the body of toxic pollutants. Scientific research has shown that these plants bind with heavy metals in the intestines helping to eliminate them from the body. The chemical makeup of seaweed is similar to human blood, and when consumed, it has a balancing, alkalizing affect. Seaweed has antibiotic properties that have been shown to be effective against penicillin-resistant bacteria.

Brown kelp improves hair health, and it's said that the thick, lustrous hair of the Japanese is due to eating brown sea vegetables that provide high mineral content.

Arame is found in dry, long, thin strands and is very sweet and mild in flavor. Arame is concentrated with iron, calcium, and potassium and is one of the richest sources of iodine. As with kombu, kelp, and hijiki, arame counteracts high blood pressure.

Hijiki has a mild flavor, and quadruples in size when hydrated. The dry pieces are thicker and shorter than arame. Of all sea vegetables, hijiki is the richest in minerals and has abundance of trace elements. Extremely high in calcium (gram for gram, fourteen times more than dairy milk), it's rich in iron and protein. Arame and Hijiki can be used interchangeably.

Wakame has a sweet flavor and is often rehydrated and added to miso soup or added into a side dish. I love making salads with it. Wakame contains anti-obesity properties and is very high in EPA, an essential fatty acid. It's rich in calcium and contains high levels of vitamins B and C. Can be substituted with dulse or arame.

Sushi Nori (sea lettuce, green laver) are the thin dark sheets used to make maki rolls. Nori is also available in flakes and works as a savory table condiment. Nori is an important part of Korean, Chinese, and Japanese cuisines. Nori is 28 percent protein, more than lentils, and is a great source of calcium, iron, manganese, fluoride, copper, and zinc. Of sea vegetables, nori is one of the highest in vitamins B-1, B-2, B-3, B-6, B-12, and the beauty vitamins A, C, and E.

Dulse is a reddish brown sea vegetable harvested from rocks where it has dried in the sun. Dulse contains about 20 percent protein, vitamins, and minerals, including calcium, potassium, magnesium, iron, and beta-carotene. Companies are starting to use dulse in skin care and cosmetic products for its beautifying and bio-available nutrient properties. Available whole and in flakes and makes a great snack and salt substitute.

Kombu (sea cabbage) is used to make a traditional soup stock called "dashi." It's usually sold dry in large strips or sheets. Choose kombu that's very dark, almost black. Kombu eases digestion, reduces blood cholesterol and hypertension, is high in iodine, potassium, calcium, and vitamins A and C and contains enzymes.

The following types of seaweeds are not used in this book, but I do stock them in my kitchen and use them in other recipes.

Spirulina is a type of blue-green algae that's 60 percent protein. It contains twelve times more digestible protein and three times more protein by weight than beef. It's rich in carotenoids, an antioxidant protecting cells from damage. Test tube studies show that spirulina boosts our immune system, protects against allergies, and has antiviral and anticancer properties. I put this in my smoothies and chocolate.

Chlorella, a great source for chlorophyll, is detoxifying and cleansing. Good for rebuilding muscle and tissues, even nerve tissue. Boosts immune system and reverses cancer. After a hard workout, I put both spirulina and chlorella into a smoothie for protein and to help repair and rebuild the muscles I've broken down.

Irish Moss (Carrageen) is used as an emulsifier and for its gelling properties. It thickens foods and produces a colorless jelly consistency. It's the vegetarian answer to gelatin, but healthier. Great to use in raw food desserts and for stiffening up raw cheezes to create a tofu texture.

SOAKING DRY SEAWEED

Dried seaweeds can be reconstituted in water, and will expand and grow. Save the soak water to use in soups.

STORAGE

Dried seaweeds can be stored in a cool, dry place for several years in an airtight container. If seaweed becomes damp, it can be dried again in your dehydrator.

INDIAN HEAD MASSAGE

Indian Head Massage has been practiced in India for over five thousand years and is based on ancient Ayurvedic medicine. It promotes relaxation, relieves eyestrain and tension headaches, increases blood circulation to the head and brain, stimulates hair growth, improves concentration, increases lymphatic flow, and helps our body detoxify.

Experts say the massage works best with an Ayurvedic medicinal oil, like bramhi or amla, but these oils may be hard to find. I use organic coconut, olive, almond, or sesame since they moisturize, condition, stimulate hair growth, and have a neutral scent. Our scalp is quick to absorb anything we put on it, so make sure to choose raw and organic.

My DIY method for Indian Head Massage is simple. I like to do this in the evening, before bed. My hair is long and thick, so I pour about a ¼ cup of oil onto my scalp. Then, massage it into my scalp and down through the ends of my hair. It feels really good to rub and touch my scalp, which otherwise gets little attention. When ready, wash with shampoo. Condition if desired. I always leave my hair to air dry. So I like to lay a towel on my pillow and then go to bed.

In addition to relaxing me, this Indian Head Massage is a natural, raw, and moisturizing "hot oil" treatment.

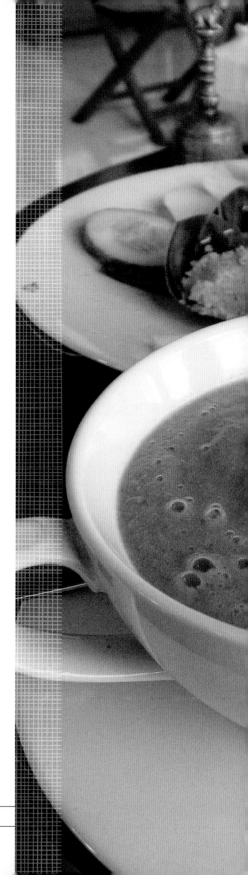

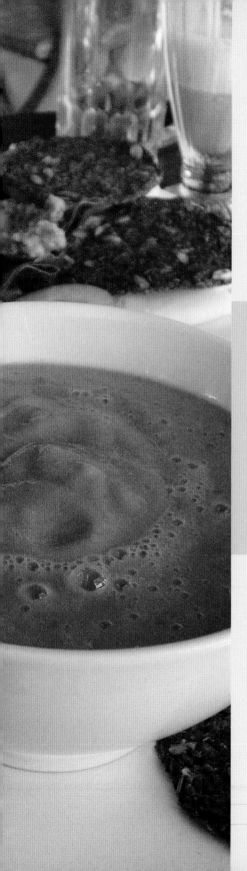

COCONUT TOMATO SOUP
Thailand

MAKES 4 SERVINGS

Tomatoes blended with creamy coconut milk, lemongrass, ginger, and garlic for the flavors of Southeast Asia. I tasted this soup while sitting on a beach in beautiful Phuket staring out over the turquoise blue lagoon. A smooth, beautifully colored soup perfect for when you want to bring the tropics home.

SOUP
2 cups chopped tomatoes (about 2 medium tomatoes)

2 tablespoons minced lemongrass

1 teaspoon chopped ginger

½ teaspoon chopped garlic

1 tablespoon agave syrup

¼ teaspoon salt

2 cups coconut milk, page 144

GARNISH
4 lime wedges

Place all soup ingredients, except for the coconut milk, into your blender. Blend smooth. Add coconut milk, blend.

To serve, transfer soup into four bowls. Garnish with lime wedge on the side.

Will keep for 3 to 4 days in fridge.

COCONUT MILK

Coconuts give us living water. It takes nine months for mineral water to be distilled through the trunk of the coconut palm before it is sealed inside the Thai baby coconut. This living water is packed full of electrolytes, providing the best way to hydrate after a hard workout. This coconut water, different from coconut milk, comes from a baby coconut whose meat is gelatinous.

When the coconut matures and becomes hairy and brown on the outside, the meat inside solidifies, and the coconut water becomes bitter. Coconut milk is traditionally made in Thailand by grating the mature, solidified coconut meat, and squeezing out the liquid.

Here're two recipes for making your own coconut milk. The first requires a mature brown coconut. The second uses dried, shredded coconut found in most grocery stores. I always prefer to use fresh, whole ingredients, but coconut milk is also found in cans in most Asian markets.

COCONUT MILK, FRESH

MAKES 1 CUP

¾ cup chopped coconut meat from mature coconut
¾ cup filtered water

Place meat and water in blender. Blend smooth. Set aside 30 minutes to steep.

Pour into strainer over a bowl, pressing pulp through strainer, and catching the milk. Squeeze remaining pulp over bowl using your hand.

Pour milk through a fine mesh strainer one more time to remove any remaining solids.

Rather than just composting, try folding remaining solids into your next batch of flax crackers, biscuits, or cookies.

COCONUT MILK USING DESICCATED COCONUT

MAKES 1 CUP

⅔ cup unsweetened shredded coconut
1 cup filtered water

Place coconut and water into blender. Set aside 30 minutes to hydrate.

Blend for one minute. Pour into a strainer over a bowl, pressing pulp through strainer, and catching the milk. Squeeze remaining pulp over bowl using your hand.

Pour milk through a fine mesh strainer one more time to remove any remaining solids.

COCONUT HOT AND SOUR SOUP WITH MIXED MARINATED MUSHROOMS

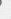

China

MAKES 4 SERVINGS

Fresh lemon and coconut flavors from coconut meat and lemongrass fill this soup. Marinated mushrooms with julienned lime leaves and lemon juice are added in for texture, protein, and flavor. And garnished with wedges of tomato and sliced carrots.

MARINADE

1 cup mixed mushrooms, like a large black oyster and/or shiitake

2 teaspoons julienned Asian lime leaves

1 tablespoon fresh lemon juice

1 tablespoon extra-virgin olive oil

GARNISH

1 cup tomato wedges (about 1 medium tomato)

¼ cup sliced carrot, cut very thinly into circles

½ cup whole snow peas

SOUP

2 cups coconut meat

1 teaspoon chopped garlic

2 tablespoons chopped lemongrass, lower stalks only

½ to 1 teaspoon fresh chile pepper, to taste

1 teaspoon sea salt

4 cups filtered water, as needed

Combine all marinade ingredients, toss to mix well. Set aside for at least 20 minutes for mushrooms to soften.

Place all soup ingredients into high-speed blender with 1 cup of water to start. Blend smooth. Then add remaining water and blend to mix well.

To serve, transfer soup into four bowls. Top with marinated mushrooms and marinade. Garnish with tomato, carrots, and snow peas.

Will keep for 1 to 2 days in fridge.

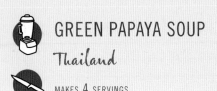

GREEN PAPAYA SOUP
Thailand

MAKES 4 SERVINGS

A soup reminiscent of a traditional *Thai Tom Kha* soup with added squares of green papaya, garnished with fresh cilantro and the flavors of lime leaf and lemongrass. Quick and easy to make in your blender.

If you can't find a green papaya, just use a ripe one instead to add a softer, sweeter flavor and brighter color.

If using a high-speed blender, it's easy to place whole ingredients into container. If using a less powerful blender, you may want to mince and chop ingredients before blending.

SOUP

2 cups coconut meat

1 teaspoon minced garlic

5 medium chopped Asian lime leaves

2 tablespoons chopped lemongrass, lower stalks only

⅓ cup coconut oil

1 teaspoon sea salt

4 cups filtered water, as needed

GARNISH

1 to 2 cups diced green papaya, as desired

2 tablespoons fresh cilantro leaves

Into blender, place all soup ingredients with just 1 cup water to start. Blend smooth. Add remaining water and blend to mix well.

Serve by transferring into four soup bowls. Add papaya and garnish with cilantro.

Will keep for 3 days in fridge.

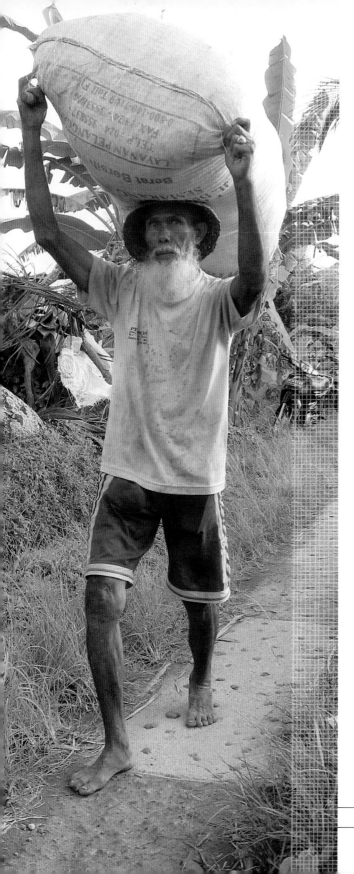

STRUCTURE AND DISCIPLINE

I've worked my entire life to create a life that's unstructured. I've gone between extremes of the office day job and combating rush-hour traffic to having a fluctuating range between waking and sleeping times each day.

Being raised by a North Korean dad, discipline was drilled into my brother and me. Practice piano and violin daily, study Korean grammar, do your homework, and follow house rules. I was enrolled in summer school every year, with little down-time ever.

I fantasized how an unstructured life would give me a sense of freedom. I'd be able to do whatever I wanted each day. I was surprised to discover people whose lives seem free and unstructured from the outside actually accomplish their success through discipline and structure. They work consistently in baby steps toward end goals for a sense of accomplishment and confidence.

Curries

Curries are made much in the same way as soups. One exception is the Jackfruit Curry, where spices are first ground together, as it's done in Indonesia, then added to a coconut milk base before vegetables are added.

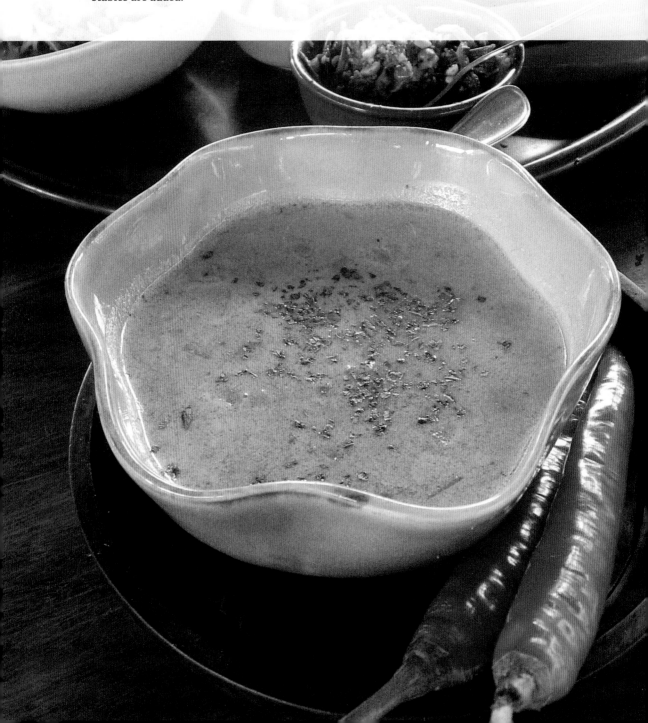

JACKFRUIT CURRY

Indonesia

MAKES 4 SERVINGS

Jackfruit smells sweet and tastes like bubblegum. Jackfruit is the largest fruit in the world to grow on a tree and is found in southern and southeast Asia, where it's a staple food and cooked in curry.

My first jackfruit curry experience was in Bali on New Year's Eve of 2010. The jackfruit looked like pork sitting in a light curry broth, so I had to keep asking to make sure it was vegan. When I ate it, I was blown away by how yummy it was. If you don't have jackfruit, replace it with 2 cups of your favorite vegetable instead.

To make this recipe, you'll first mortar or process a batch of chile paste and then mix it into coconut milk with wine, optional, to make the curry broth. Then, add jackfruit, basil, and cashews to the broth to finish before serving.

CHILE PASTE

3 sliced spring onions

1 fresh red chile, to taste

4 whole Asian lime leaves, fresh or frozen

1 teaspoon minced garlic

1 tablespoon lemon or lime juice

½ cup fresh basil leaves

2 tablespoon coconut oil

2 tablespoons soy sauce

1 tablespoon agave or maple syrup

BROTH

1 cup coconut milk, page 144

2 tablespoons white wine, optional

VEGETABLES

2 cups diced jackfruit

¼ cup chiffonade basil leaves

¼ cup whole cashews

Process paste ingredients together in a food processor. Or, use a mortar and pestle to first pound dry ingredients, then add wet ingredients and mix well.

To make your curry broth, mix together paste with coconut milk and wine, if using.

To serve, place jackfruit into four serving bowls. Scoop on curry and top with basil leaves and cashews.

Will keep for several days in the fridge.

YELLOW COCONUT CURRY VEGETABLES

India

MAKES 4 SERVINGS

Inspired by an Indian curry, coconut milk is mixed with the flavors of coriander, cumin, ginger, and garlic, with a bit of spicy cayenne. Serve this yellow curry with mixed vegetables and garnish with fragrant lemongrass and basil.

CURRY SAUCE

½ cup liquid coconut oil

½ cup Coconut Milk, page 144

1 tablespoon coriander powder

1 tablespoon cumin powder

1 tablespoon turmeric powder

2 teaspoons grated ginger

2 teaspoons minced garlic

¼ teaspoon sea salt

Pinch cayenne powder, to taste

VEGETABLES

1 cup seeded and sliced red bell pepper
   (about 1 medium pepper)

1 cup tomato wedges (about 1 medium tomato)

½ cup sliced green beans, cut into 2-inch
   lengths

½ cup crumbled cauliflower

½ cup corn kernels

¼ cup mung bean sprouts

GARNISH

1 tablespoon finely chopped lemongrass

½ cup lightly chopped loose basil leaves

"Deep-Fried" shallots, page 206, optional

Place all curry sauce ingredients in a bowl or blender and mix well. If using blender, pour sauce into mixing bowl. Add vegetables and toss to mix well. You can enjoy immediately, or set aside to marinate and soften for at least 30 minutes.

To serve, transfer to serving bowls. Garnish by sprinkling on lemongrass, basil, and shallots, if using.

Vegetables in curry will keep for 2 days in fridge.

ORANGE COCONUT CURRY SAUCE

India

MAKES 4 SERVINGS

A light sauce with the flavors of coconut and orange. Psyllium seed helps thicken and adds fiber and volume in this recipe. Psyllium has a distinct flavor, so use sparingly. Start with 1 tablespoon, mix well, and set curry aside for a few minutes to thicken. Add additional powder slowly, ½ to 1 teaspoon at a time, if you want your curry sauce thicker, tasting to make sure the psyllium flavor's not over-powering the recipe. Psyllium is available at natural food stores.

Coconut oil is solid at room temperature. To liquefy your coconut oil, place bottle into a bowl of hot water. Oil will melt. Pour off ¼ cup and use in recipe.

Add your favorite vegetables to make a vegetable curry. Or, try this curry as the base to a soup, or even serve as a dipping sauce.

3 cups Coconut Milk, page 144

½ cup fresh orange juice

⅓ cup liquid coconut oil

2 tablespoons mild yellow curry powder

3 tablespoons minced yellow onion

1 tablespoon psyllium seed powder, as needed, as thickener

3 teaspoons orange zest

½ teaspoon minced garlic, from about 1 clove

3 tablespoons fresh cilantro leaves, as garnish

Place all ingredients, except cilantro, into a mixing bowl. Whisk to mix well.

SERVING SUGGESTIONS: *Add 2 to 3 cups of your favorite vegetables and toss to coat and mix well. Set aside for 15 minutes or longer to marinate before serving. Or scoop 1 cup curry into four soup bowls and top with shredded greens or vegetables. Garnish with cilantro before serving.*

CURRY SAUCE WITH RAISINS

Hawaii

MAKES 4 SERVINGS

This recipe was inspired by a vegetable curry I tasted in Oahu. It was light, fresh, and spicy. Adjust the curry powder to your liking to adjust the heat levels in this curry. Use this curry with your favorite vegetables.

2 tablespoons chopped yellow onion

½ teaspoon minced garlic

1 cup cored, peeled, and chopped apple, from about 1 small apple, any type

3 tablespoons extra-virgin olive oil

1 tablespoon curry powder

1 teaspoon minced ginger

3 cups Coconut Milk, page 144

½ cup raisins, any type

Place all ingredients, except the Coconut Milk and raisins, into your high-speed blender. Starting with half the Coconut Milk, blend smooth, then add the remaining milk and blend to mix well. Add raisins and set aside to soak and reconstitute for 10 to 15 minutes.

Serving ideas: Add 2 to 3 cups of your favorite vegetables and toss to coat and mix well. Set aside for 15 minutes or longer to marinate before serving. Or scoop 1 cup curry into four soup bowls and top with shredded greens or vegetables.

RENDANG CURRY

Indonesia

MAKES 4 SERVINGS

Rendang is an Indonesian "dry" curry that's typically simmered down into a very flavorful sauce that sticks onto vegetables and meats. So this is a curry you'll want to massage onto your favorite vegetables.

Thai red chiles are spicy, so adjust levels to create the heat index you prefer. You can use a mortar and pestle to pound the dry ingredients together first, or just place everything into your high speed blender and whip this curry up in a few seconds.

CURRY

2 tablespoons finely chopped lemongrass

2 tablespoons chopped yellow onion

½ teaspoon minced garlic, about 1 clove

1 teaspoon grated ginger

½ to 1 Thai red chile, to taste

1 tablespoon brown rice or agave syrup,
    or stevia powder, to taste

1 tablespoon Nama Shoyu or tamari

1 tablespoon coriander powder

1 tablespoon cumin powder

1 teaspoon cinnamon powder

1 cup Coconut Milk, page 144

GARNISH

2 tablespoons cilantro, or coriander, leaves

2 tablespoons dried shredded coconut

To make your curry, you can use your mortar and pestle to pound your dry ingredients and spices first. Then add liquids to mix well, whisking in the coconut milk last. Or, simply place all curry ingredients into blender and blend to mix smooth.

Use curry to massage about 2 to 3 cups of your favorite vegetables like cauliflower and broccoli florets, peas, corn, and diced zucchini. Set aside to marinate for 15 or more minutes before serving.

To serve, scoop vegetables onto a serving dish, and garnish with cilantro and shredded coconut.

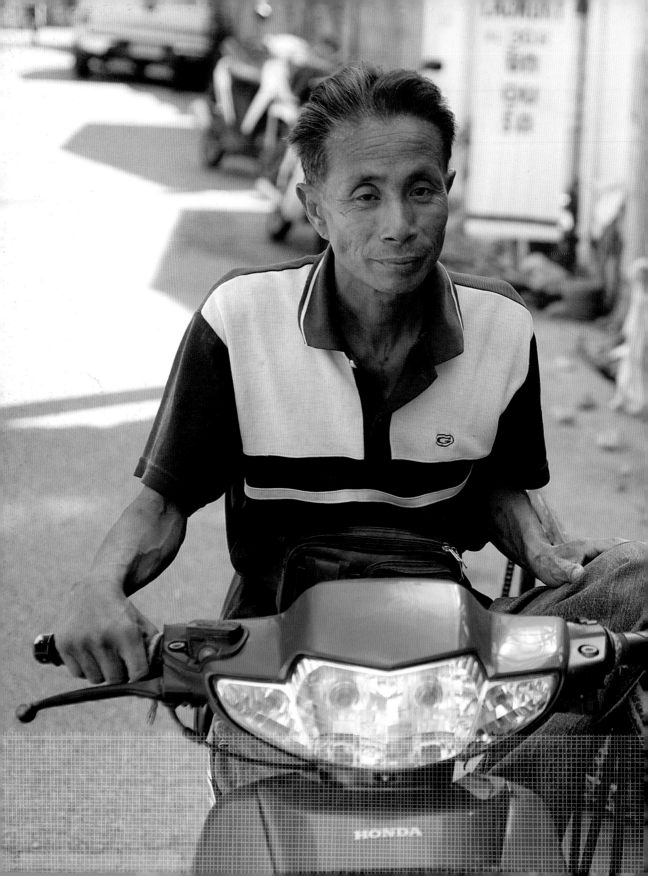

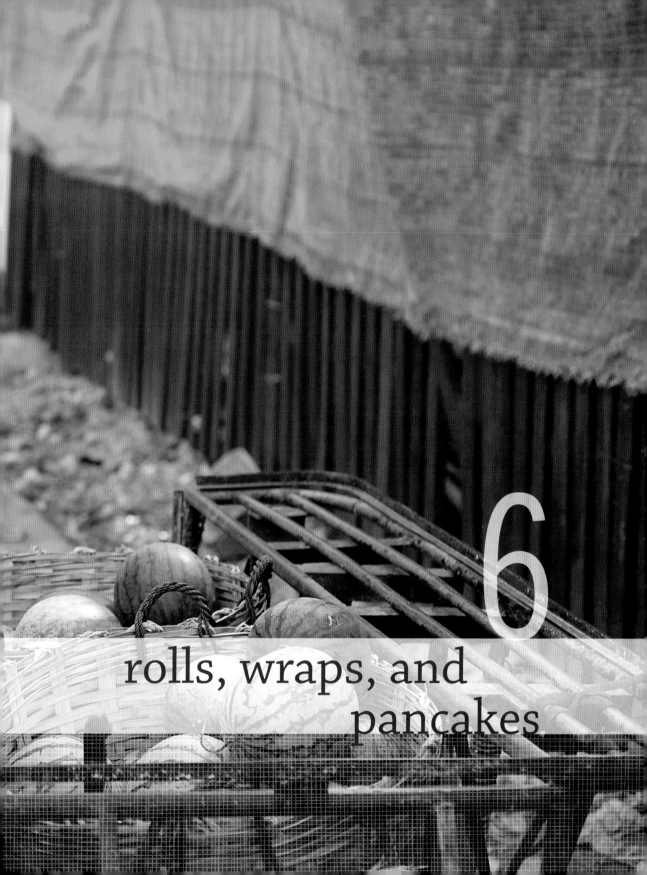

6

rolls, wraps, and
pancakes

Physical Fitness

A balanced raw-food diet provides the trillions of cells in our body with nutrients they need to super-perform. With the right nutrients, our brains function more clearly, it's easier to make the right decisions, we become stronger and healthier, and we feel happier. In addition to good nutrition, it's also important to move, stretch, and strengthen our bodies through exercise.

Fitness includes more than just cardio training. A combination of stretching and yoga for flexibility and lengthening, cardio exercise and sweating for heart health, and building strength for strong bones and muscles all contribute to our level of fitness. Fun and variety in our workouts stimulate our brain, keep us on our toes, and help us avoid getting bored with doing the same thing day after day.

Raw foods are nutrient-dense and easy to digest, making them great fuel for weight loss, building lean muscle mass, strengthening, boosting our metabolism and immune system . . . all while alleviating overall stress levels, contributing to a long life.

WEIGHT LOSS

Sometimes, I want to decrease body fat and get leaner, and end up actually gaining weight from muscle mass while losing body fat. Instead of measuring my fitness by reading the scale, I strive to be strong, powerful, and healthy.

The speed of our metabolism can depend on our genetics, muscle mass, and age (our metabolisms slow down after forty). One of the keys to longevity is maintaining a constant body weight throughout life, instead of putting on more and more pounds as we age. To lose one pound in weight, you have to subtract 3,500 calories from your diet.

In Korea, some women won't exercise because they don't want muscle definition, and they'll starve themselves to be skinny. My mom was really thin for most of my life. It was stressful for her to take care of my ill father plus raise my brother and me on her own after Dad passed on to the next level. Today, Mom's about 20 pounds heavier, but stronger and healthier for it. She works out daily at home or at the gym lifting weights, going to dance class, walking, or just stretching.

There have been times when I've restricted my calories so much, I didn't have the strength to push through a hard workout nor did my body have sufficient building blocks for recovery post-workout. I would feel run-down and tired. It can take up to 2 weeks for our body to fully recover after a hard workout. Without sufficient recovery time, stress increases, causing our adrenal glands to produce too much cortisol. This in turn causes weight gain around the midsection, a depressed immune system, and insomnia, to name a few ill effects.

To keep myself fit and healthy (rather than looking at numbers on the scale), I work to build vitality and strength. It's a delicate balance between training, resting, and surprisingly, being careful not to over-train.

A SIMPLE EQUATION

Weight loss is a calorie-in and calorie-out equation. Notice that sweet fruits and fats have the highest amount of calories compared to vegetables and limit eating them if you want to shed pounds. Hydration is also essential for a healthy, vital body, so drink plenty of water. Eating more protein will help increase your muscle mass—and this will help to boost your metabolism.

Limiting higher-calorie foods like sweet fruits, nuts, oils, and fats is one step; cutting out allergens like wheat, dairy, soy, and peanuts, which cause inflammation and swelling, can also help. Instead, eat more greens like wheatgrass juice, spinach, kale, sea vegetables including spirulina and chlorella. And, eat more protein from hemp and buckwheat groats. I can't stress the importance of hydration enough. Coconut water, green smoothies, and water kefir (a probiotic drink that strengthens our immune system and builds healthy intestinal flora) are all electrolyte-laden beverages. Supplement with maca root powder for its adrenal-supporting benefits. I talk about maca in *Ani's Raw Food Desserts* as being an adaptogen that strengthens our body's stress center, namely our adrenal glands, enabling us to take on more stress before it runs us down or makes us ill. The energy it provides us is not fake, as with caffeine, but rather, we feel stronger because we are stronger. Maca is popular with athletes who want to power up without tricking the body into thinking it has energy it's borrowing, as with caffeine.

EAT MORE WATER

Fresh raw foods contain naturally distilled water. Eat more fruits and veggies and drink more water. The body needs water to burn calories. Studies have found adults who drink eight or more glasses of water a day burn more calories than those who drink only four.

SNACK MORE

Eating more frequently by enjoying a snack every 3 hours or so will keep your metabolism revved up. Eating large meals less frequently trains your metabolism to slow down. It's as if your metabolism is a furnace. You want to keep stoking the furnace every few hours to keep the fire burning evenly, rather than waiting until the fire is almost out, then adding more wood to get the fire going again. You'll burn more calories over the entire day by eating smaller, frequent snacks.

ADD SPICE

Chile contains capsaicin, which is the ingredient in diet pills that speeds up our metabolism. Adding heat to your food can boost your metabolism up to 23 percent. Studies show the effect only lasts about 30 to 60 minutes, but eaten frequently, it adds up.

MORE PROTEIN

I never worried about my protein intake in the past, but now I realize my body needs more protein as it ages. Protein is what builds muscle along with the collagen in our skin to keep us looking youthful, longer. It takes the body more energy, up to double the calories, to burn protein. So eating more protein will boost your metabolism.

AVOID DIETS AND FASTING

Eating fewer than 1,000 calories a day may help you drop pounds in the near term, but most of that loss is muscle. When we starve ourselves, our body cannibalizes our muscle to feed itself. This lowers our muscle mass and slows down our metabolism, which means your body will burn fewer, not more calories. Once you start eating normally again, you will gain weight faster than before the fast. I know this from personal experience with different types of fasts over the course of 8 years.

It's possible to eat a lot of food by paying attention to what you're eating. The most calories come from fat and sugar. One cup of orange has about 90 calories while a cup of spinach has only 7. So eat up greens and vegetables and moderate in the case of fruits, sweeteners, fats, and oils.

AVOID ALLERGENS

Avoid common allergens and food intolerances to wheat, dairy, soy, and peanuts. Eating these foods commonly causes an allergy reaction in the body, which includes inflammation, swelling, and bloating. Raw foods do not use these common allergens, are cleansing and detoxing, and work to decrease inflammation. The result is a tighter and leaner body.

INCREASED ENERGY

We all know exercise is good for us. Exercise does produce free radicals and increases our metabolic rate, which makes us age more quickly. However, studies show people who exercise regularly live longer than sedentary people, regardless of their weight. And, exercise gets our blood pumped with oxygen, pushing out stagnated blood and toxins. The right exercise in the right amounts gives us energy and makes us stronger, while lack of exercise or over-exercise depletes our health.

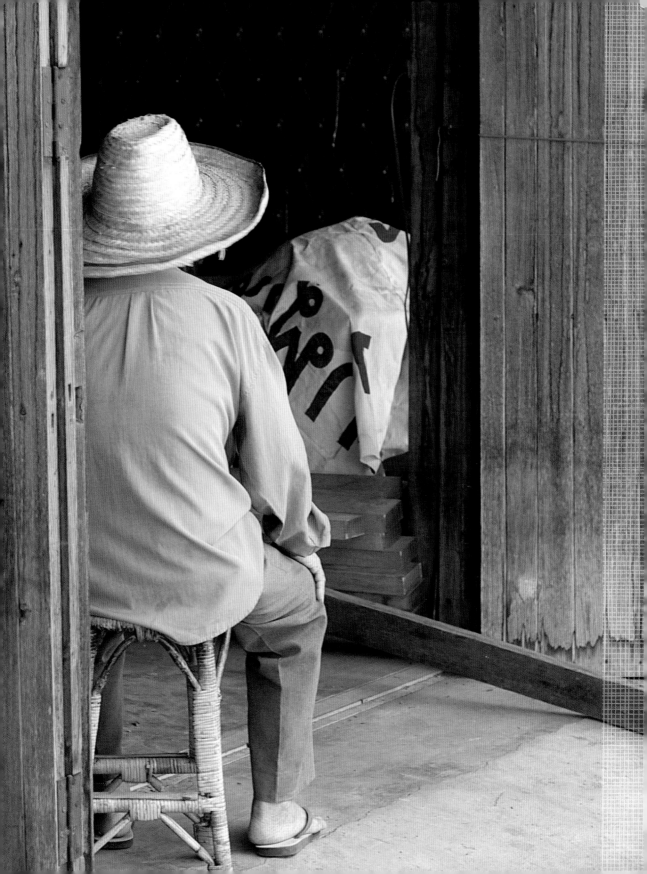

ASIAN TRADITIONS AND PHYSICAL FITNESS

Heart disease, obesity, diabetes, and many cancers continue to rise in America, but are much less common in Asian countries. Physical activity in Asia blends spirituality with fitness, as with tai chi, and the Asian diet is fresher and healthier. Research has found the average Chinese adult eats half as much fat and one-third less protein than the average American. The Chinese diet is made up of mostly grains, fruits, and vegetables. Meat, if used, is an accompaniment or side dish, never a main. Fish and green tea's antioxidant benefits have also been found to contribute to the healthier Asian lifestyle. However, rates of obesity and traditionally Western illness like diabetes are on the rise in the east—because we've exported our Standard American Diet (SAD).

Studies of "longevity clusters" show that the world's longest-living people are mostly in Asia. Check out Dr. T. Colin Campbell's *The China Study* (2006). It's based on twenty years of research among Cornell University, Oxford University, and the Chinese Academy of Preventative Medicine. "People who ate the most animal-based foods got the most chronic disease. . . . People who ate the most plant-based foods were the healthiest and tended to avoid chronic disease. These results could not be ignored," said Dr. Campbell. He recommends avoiding processed foods (like vegan junk foods) and sticking to a whole-food, fresh, plant-based diet for optimal health and longevity.

To increase energy, eat fruits, sea vegetables including spirulina and chlorella, and maca. Maca is an adaptogen, strengthens our adrenals, and increases our body's ability to handle stress. It makes us stronger, naturally, without caffeine. Hydrate with fruit smoothies, coconut water, and water kefir.

STRENGTH BUILDING

Weight-bearing exercise is important for maintaining healthy, strong bones. I love pumping iron and flexing my muscles. It's fun and feels great. And, I find it encouraging to watch myself grow stronger over time. Asians naturally have a lower bone density, and the last time I was tested a decade ago, I was diagnosed with osteopenia, meaning I had lower than normal peak bone mineral density (BMD). That was one reason I started a regular weight-lifting routine, to help make my bones stronger.

Muscle feeds on fat, and the more muscle mass we have, the higher our resting metabolic rate is. A pound of muscle will burn about 6 calories a day, while a pound of fat burns just 2 calories. So it's important to activate our muscles daily to increase our daily metabolic rate. I lift heavy weights one to two days a week.

To build muscle, you need protein from greens, wheatgrass, sea vegetables—like kelp, wakame, nori, spirulina, and chlorella—hemp protein, quinoa, buckwheat, maca, and sprouts. Hydrate with coconut water, protein smoothies, and water kefir.

OSTEOPOROSIS

Amino acids from animal protein leaches calcium from our bones to neutralize the acid. In America, our diet is high in dairy and animal products. The media sells dairy as building healthy bones when it actually contributes to osteoporosis. In Asia, the "cheese" and "milk" come from soy instead of dairy in the form of tofu and soy milk. Fewer animal products and less meat are eaten in Asia than in America. And, there are very low rates of osteoporosis.

Cornell University researchers T. Colin Campbell and Banoo Parpia found that eating less meat does more to reduce the risk of osteoperosis than increasing calcium intake because animal protein, including dairy products, leaches more calcium from bones than is ingested.

"This phenomenon could explain why Americans, who ingest much higher levels of calcium, have much higher rates of osteoporosis and hip fractures compared with many Chinese and other Asians who consume few dairy products and ingest low amounts of calcium," Campbell said. Hip fractures in the United States are approximately five times more frequent than in China. His studies have found that countries with the highest calcium intakes have the highest bone fracture rates while low-calcium vegetarian diets have increased bone density. In addition, casein (the protein in daily milk) contributes to high cholesterol levels in the West while also significantly enhancing tumor growth.

"Vegetarians obtain plenty of calcium and appear to have higher rates of bone density, which predispose them to lower rates of osteoporosis," said Campbell. He also states that Americans will not reduce their rates of cancer, cardiovascular disease, and other chronic, degenerative diseases until they shift from an animal-based diet to a plant-based diet. Animal-based diets are high in fat and low in fiber while plant-based diets are generally low in fat and high in fiber. Plant-based diets have other beneficial substances like antioxidants, which combat free-radical damage and help prevent cancer. Campbell's studies also show daily physical exercise help to protect bone health in both pre- and postmenopausal women.

Don't buy the hype that dairy is the main source of calcium. There are plenty of amazing, great-tasting, plant-based sources of calcium: sea vegetables are a great source, as are sesame seeds, tahini, and dark leafy greens.

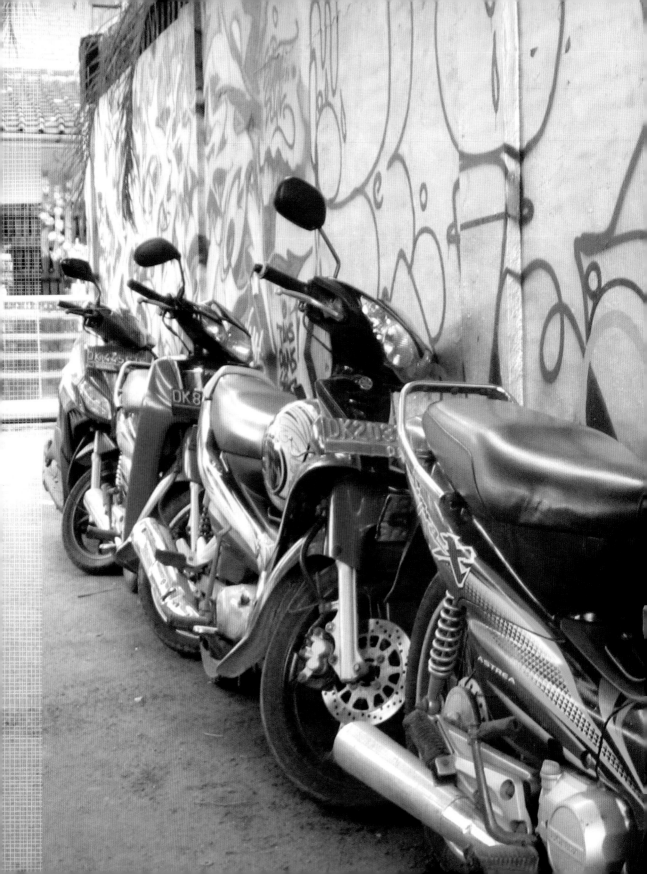

CARDIO AND HEART HEALTH

Working out at higher intensity levels increases our metabolic rate, and the boost lasts longer than for moderate workouts. Include bursts of running in with your walking. I used to be a cardio freak, but as I age, my joints aren't as happy. Instead, shorter and more intense workouts work better for me and my joints. It's critical to build a strong heart that will pump oxygen and blood powerfully. That means it can beat less frequently, which decreases wear and tear, and it will last longer.

I've started taking a new approach to incorporate a day for recovery between hard workouts to contribute to my longevity and overall vitality. Rather than lifting weights and doing cardio at the gym, I may choose to walk or ride my bike to dinner, or just stretch, do some yoga, or do breath work instead.

To boost your endurance workouts, fuel up with maca, fruits like banana and dates for immediate glucose energy, buckwheat, quinoa, hemp protein, wheatgrass, and sea vegetables. Hydrate with coconut water, fruit smoothies, and water kefir.

FLEXIBILILTY

Stretching and lengthening our bodies is just as important as weight-bearing exercise and cardio. Remember how flexible you were as a child? We're meant to stay that flexible; unfortunately, over time, many of us become less active and lose our flexibility.

Yoga is a long-standing Eastern tradition (and a significant part of Ayurveda) that's only recently become popular in the West. Yoga is a great way to stretch; consistency and a daily practice will increase flexibility over time. Yogis believe our youth is defined by the flexibility in our spine.

To increase flexibility, avoid foods that cause inflammation and swelling like soy, corn, wheat, dairy, meat, processed foods, flour, refined sugar, salt, carbohydrates, and toxic chemicals like artificial flavors, colors, pesticides, herbicides, and genetically modified foods. Instead, enjoy more hemp protein, spirulina, chlorella, maca, fruits, vegetables, and anti-inflammatory foods like ginger and turmeric. Sulfur improves elasticity and flexibility. My favorite fruit, durian, is a great source of sulfur and MSM (methylsulfonylmethane), which is sold as a supplement for decreasing pain and inflammation. Hydrate with coconut water, fruit smoothies, and water kefir.

Rolls, Wraps, and Pancakes

Rolls, wraps, and pancakes all make great handheld treats; they are also beautiful on a platter when eco entertaining, for a romantic dinner for two, for picnics, and when traveling.

Rolls and wraps are traditionally made by wrapping ingredients like a spinach curry inside a rice paper wrapper, but instead, I use a coconut dosa wrapper. Spring rolls can be wrapped with thinly sliced cucumber, then stuffed with fresh thai herbs. Pancakes are made with a batter of baby coconut meat with corn or scallions and your favorite vegetables mixed in and served with a spicy and salty dipping sauce. Unlike the sweet pancakes popular in America, pancakes in Asia are savory and are popular in Indian, Korean, and Vietnamese cuisine. Pancakes are beautiful as part of any meal and are an easy travel food, too. Traditionally, pancakes are made with rice flour, but I use coconut meat as the base in my raw recipes.

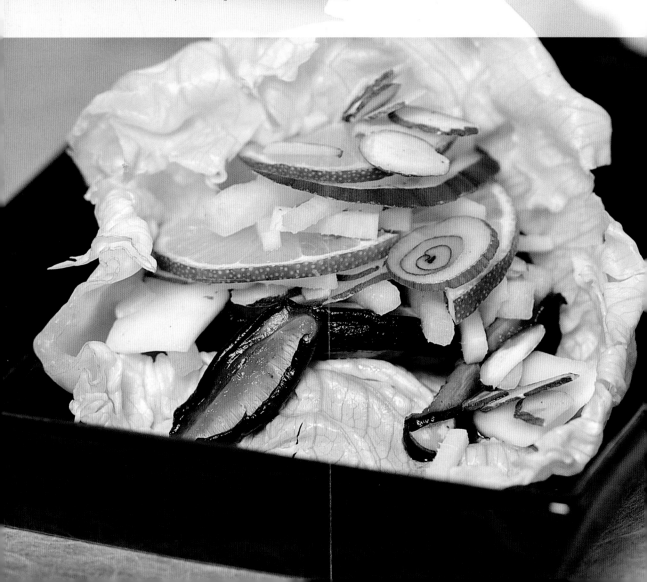

ICEBERG LETTUCE WRAPS WITH MOCK TAMARIND SAUCE
Thailand

MAKES 4 SERVINGS

Light, fresh, and easy lettuce cups filled with tart citrus, spicy ginger, and the crunch of slivered almonds. In this recipe I use jicama instead of water chestnut for a similar mouth feel and add pieces of fresh coconut meat, too. Serve with a sweet and tart Tamarind Sauce.

MARINATED MUSHROOMS

½ cup sliced shiitake mushrooms

1 teaspoon extra-virgin olive oil

1 teaspoon Nama Shoyu

FILLING

½ cup julienned jicama

½ cup diced Thai baby coconut meat

¼ cup thinly sliced red onion

¼ cup slivered almonds

¼ cup julienned ginger

1 lime, thinly sliced

WRAPS

8 small iceberg leaves, which will act as lettuce cups

SAUCE

1 batch Tamarind Sauce, page 166, or Mock Tamarind Sauce, page 167

Place mushrooms in a bowl with oil and Nama Shoyu. Toss to mix well, then set aside for at least 20 minutes to soften and marinate. Squeeze out all excess liquid before using.

Assemble your wraps by scooping the marinated mushrooms into the bottom of each cup. Then, layer each filling ingredient into your eight wrapper cups. Drizzle on your Tamarind Sauce.

Serve on a platter or on individual plates with a side of Tamarind Sauce.

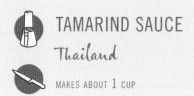

TAMARIND SAUCE
Thailand

MAKES ABOUT 1 CUP

Tamarind is also known as the Indian date. The fruit is tart and sits encased in a long, brown pod. Inside the pod is the soft, brown pulp with hard, smooth seeds. The pulp is the fruit and is rich in vitamins C and B, fiber, potassium, magnesium, and antioxidants and helps the body digest food. Tamarind is used in India, Jamaica, and Aruba, typically mixed with sugar in sauces and candies. I love eating tamarind whole, by the pod, fresh.

It takes a lot of energy to scrape and collect enough of the fruit off the seeds. If you are using fresh, you'll need to soak the tamarind overnight. You don't have to use fresh tamarind; you can start with packaged paste, which you can find at Asian markets. Usually, the fruit is heated to separate it from the seeds, so the paste will most likely be cooked. Otherwise, to skip tamarind, try the raw mock recipe on the next page.

¼ cup tamarind pulp, ripe and seedless, or tamarind paste

1 cup filtered water

1 tablespoon agave syrup

½ teaspoon cumin seeds

1 tablespoon chopped mint leaves

Soak tamarind in water overnight. The next day, mash pulp into the soaking water.

Into blender, place tamarind mash, agave syrup, and cumin. Blend smooth.

Serve chilled and sprinkled with mint.

Will keep for 4 days in fridge.

MOCK TAMARIND SAUCE
Thailand

MAKES ABOUT ½ CUP

An alternative tamarind-inspired sauce made using ingredients that are already staples in a raw kitchen, like dates, prunes, and apricots.

1 tablespoon chopped dates

1 tablespoon chopped prunes

1 tablespoon chopped dried apricots

⅓ cup filtered water, warm

1 tablespoon lemon juice

1 tablespoon agave syrup

½ teaspoon cumin seeds

1 tablespoon chopped mint leaves

Into small bowl, place dates, prunes, and apricots. Pour the filtered water over to cover fruit completely. Let stand an hour, until softened.

Place fruit with liquid, lemon juice, agave syrup, and cumin into blender. Blend to a thick paste.

Serve chilled and sprinkled with mint.

Will keep for 4 days in fridge.

MINT CHUTNEY
India

MAKES ABOUT 1 CUP

A beautiful green cilantro and mint chutney with spice from jalapeño pepper, bite from ginger, and pungency from garlic. Serve as accompaniment with any dish, especially dosas and samosas.

4 teaspoons garlic, about 8 cloves

1 tablespoon grated ginger

1 bunch cilantro, about 2 cups

2 tablespoons mint leaves, about 10

3 tablespoon Nama Shoyu or Tamari

2 teaspoons apple cider vinegar

1 or 2 jalapeño peppers, to taste

Place ingredients into a small blender, and blend smooth.

Will keep for a couple of weeks or more in fridge.

SAMOSAS WITH TOMATO DAL AND MOCK TAMARIND SAUCE

India

MAKES 4 SERVINGS

A samosa is traditionally a pocket that's deep-fried and filled with curried potatoes, peas, and onions. This wrapper-free raw version is inspired by the spices and ingredients of a fried samosa blended into a patty similar to a falafel.

Cashews and flax are processed into a thick batter, with spices. Then filling ingredients like broccoli, peas, and corn are added for texture, color, and flavor. Pyramids are shaped and dehydrated. Serve with Tomato Dal and Mock Tamarind Sauce.

If you don't have a dehydrator yet, you can use your oven on the lowest setting to dry your samosas. To keep it more on the raw side, try propping open your oven door with a chopstick. I know, it's hardly eco green, but I'm hoping this may inspire you to acquire a dehydrator.

BATTER

1¼ cup cashews

¼ cup golden flax meal

¼ teaspoon sea salt

1½ teaspoons curry powder

½ cup diced zucchini

1 teaspoon grated ginger

½ teaspoon minced garlic

2 tablespoons fresh lemon juice

2 tablespoons filtered water, as needed

FILLING

¼ cup chopped broccoli

¼ cup chopped cilantro

3 tablespoons peas

2 tablespoons chopped yellow onion

2 tablespoons corn kernels

GARNISH

1 batch Tomato Dal, page 169

1 batch Tamarind Sauce, page 166, or
    Mock Tamarind Sauce, page 167

Into food processor, place cashews, flax, salt, and curry powder. Grind into powder. Add the remaining batter ingredients and mix well, adding just enough water to create a thick batter.

Next, add filling ingredients into food processor. Pulse lightly only to mix filling evenly throughout the batter. Do not over-process.

Scoop out the batter with filling from food processor, and form four pyramids. Place onto one dehydrator tray.

Dehydrate pyramids for 4 to 6 hours at 104°F, until desired consistency.

To serve, scoop Tomato Dal into bottom of four bowls or dishes. Transfer a samosa onto each. Enjoy immediately with Mock Tamarind sauce.

Samosa will keep for 4 days in fridge.

SERVING SUGGESTION: *Serve with Mint Chutney, page 000*

TOMATO DAL

India

MAKES 4 SERVINGS

Traditionally, dal is a legume-based Indian dish. My dal uses almonds, sunflower seeds, tomato, and cucumber processed together to make a creamy and chunky "dal," without the lentils. Flavors of cumin and curry add an authentic Indian flair.

¼ cup almonds

¼ cup sunflower seeds

1 cup diced tomato

1 cup diced cucumber

¾ teaspoon cumin

½ teaspoon curry

2 tablespoons chopped sun dried tomatoes

¼ cup extra-virgin olive oil

¼ teaspoon sea salt

In a food processor, process almonds and sunflower seeds into small pieces. Add tomato, cucumber, cumin, curry, and sundried tomatoes. Process to mix well. Add oil and salt and process to mix.

Will keep for 3 days in fridge.

SUMMER ROLLS WITH GINGER "PEANUT" SAUCE

Vietnam

MAKES 4 SERVINGS

Fresh rolls of thinly sliced cucumber wrappers are filled with kelp noodles, sprouts, mint, basil, cilantro, and chile then served with a ginger "peanut" dipping sauce. If you don't have kelp noodles on hand, substitute with spiralized zucchini noodles or shredded carrots.

FILLING

1 cup shredded Boston lettuce leaves

1 cup kelp noodles, cut into 3-inch lengths

½ cup mung bean sprouts, rinsed

3 tablespoons mint leaves

3 tablespoons basil or Thai basil leaves

3 tablespoons cilantro leaves

1 teaspoon Thai hot pepper, serrano pepper, or other small hot chile pepper, seeded and julienned

WRAPPER

2 cucumbers, sliced very thin lengthwise, using mandoline slicer

SAUCE

1 batch Ginger "Peanut" Sauce, page 173

Place filling ingredients into bowls and arrange on your table or countertop.

To assemble rolls, place a strip of cucumber onto a flat surface, like a cutting board. Layer a scant 2 tablespoons lettuce and 2 tablespoons noodles at one end of the cucumber, followed by 1 tablespoon bean sprouts, 1 teaspoon mint leaves, 1 teaspoon basil, 1 teaspoon cilantro, 2 pieces of pepper. Place four cucumber sticks to either side of your noodle, herb, and spice pile.

Roll fillings up inside cucumber strip diagonally. Place in a container. Repeat.

To serve, transfer rolls onto a serving plate or four dishes. Serve with a side of Ginger "Peanut" Sauce for dipping.

These are best eaten immediately, but they will keep in fridge for 1 day.

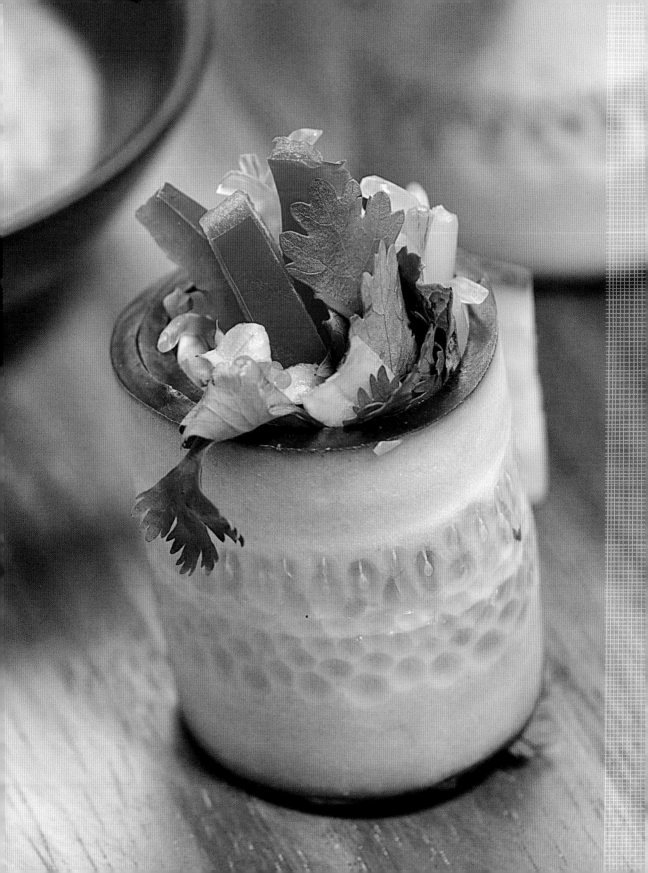

RITUALS

Having some sort of structure to the day helps provide us with a sense of purpose, gives us something to look forward to and increases our level of happiness. It can be as simple as waking up to read the morning news over a cup of tea, meditating, or going on a daily lunchtime run.

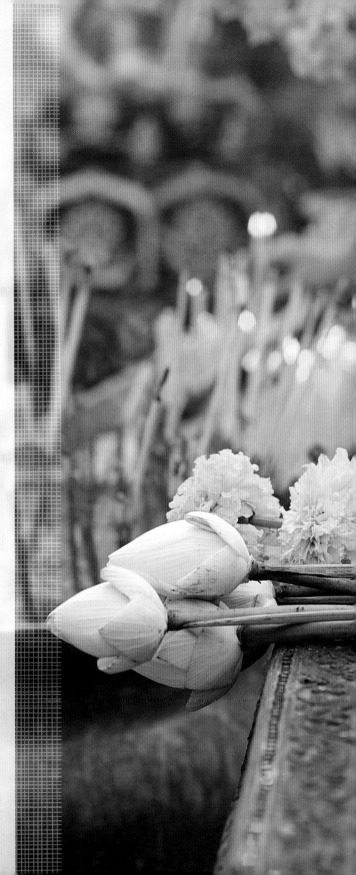

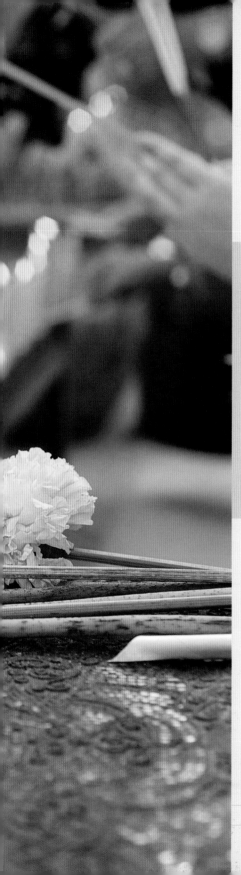

GINGER "PEANUT" SAUCE

Vietnam

MAKES ABOUT 1 CUP

Raw peanuts don't taste very good, so this sweet and savory Thai peanut sauce–inspired dip is made with almond
butter, coconut water, ginger, and lime zest.

SAUCE

¾ cup almond butter

¼ cup lemon juice

2 tablespoons Nama Shoyu

2 tablespoons agave syrup

1 teaspoon grated ginger

½ teaspoon minced garlic

½ cup coconut water, or filtered water, as desired

GARNISH

2 tablespoons lightly chopped cilantro

2 teaspoons lime zest

In blender, place all sauce ingredients. Blend smooth, adding just
enough water for desired dipping consistency.

To serve, scoop into small bowl. Sprinkle on cilantro and lime zest
before serving.

Will keep for 5 days in fridge.

RENDANG CURRY–FILLED SAMOSAS

India

MAKES 4 SERVINGS

This recipe follows more of a traditional Indian-style wrapped samosa, but using sweet Pineapple Coconut Wrappers and filled with Indonesian-inspired Rendang curried vegetables.

FILLING

½ cup tiny florets cauliflower and broccoli

¼ cup diced zucchini, cut into tiny blocks

1 batch Rendang Curry, page 153

WRAPPER

½ batch Coconut Wrappers, page 178, or Pineapple Coconut Wrappers, page 179, cut into eight rectangles
    (cut one 14 x 14-inch sheet into four rows and two columns to form eight rectangles)

DIPPING SAUCE

1 batch Tamarind Sauce, page 166, and/or

1 batch Mint Chutney, page 167, and/or

1 batch Tomato Mango Sambal, page 229

To make filling, massage cauliflower, broccoli, and zucchini with curry to coat very well. Set aside for 15 to 20 minutes or longer to marinate.

To make samosas, place one rectangular wrapper onto a flat surface. Place about a tablespoon of filling on left side of wrapper about an inch in from the left edge. Fold left edge up and over the filling to meet top edge to form a perfect triangle. Seal top edge together. Flip remaining wrapper over the filling to form triangle and to seal in filling.

Place stuffed samosas onto a dehydrator tray, and dry at 104°F for 3 to 4 hours, or to desired consistency.

To serve, place on serving dish with your favorite dipping sauces. Best enjoyed immediately.

VEGETABLE PAKORA
India

MAKES 4 SERVINGS

Pakoras are Indian vegetable fritters traditionally made with a spicy chickpea flour. I like using cauliflower and onions the best, but you can use your favorite vegetable cut into 1-inch chunks. Vegetables are coated in an Indian-spiced Coconut Wrapper batter, then dehydrated.

BATTER

1 batch Coconut Wrappers, page 178

¼ teaspoon chile powder, to taste

1 teaspoon coriander powder

1 teaspoon cumin seeds

½ teaspoon minced garlic

FILLING

2 cups vegetables, like cauliflower florets, mushrooms (halved), onions (sliced into rings),
bell peppers (diced)

To make your batter, mix together all ingredients well.

To make pakora, dip vegetables into batter and place onto a lined dehydrator tray. Dry at 104°F for 6 to 8 hours, until desired consistency.

To serve, place on serving dish. Serve with your favorite dipping sauces, or even catsup, see "Rice" with Catsup and Vegetables in Coconut Wrapper, page 189.

CORN FRITTERS WITH A HOT AND SOUR CUCUMBER DIPPING SAUCE

Indonesia

MAKES 4 SERVINGS

This is a popular Indonesian street food called *Perkedel Jagung*, a celebration of corn accompanied by ginger, garlic, and coriander and served with a cool, sweet, and spicy dipping sauce called *Saus Lado*. Garlic is left in larger pieces to avoid sticking to your fritter when dipping.

If you don't have a dehydrator yet, you can use your oven on the lowest setting to dry your fritters. To keep it as raw as possible, prop open your oven door with a chopstick. This method is hardly eco green, but I'm hoping you may be inspired to acquire a dehydrator.

DIPPING SAUCE

2 fresh red Thai chiles, seeded and finely sliced

1 clove garlic, sliced into four pieces

1 tablespoon seeded, minced cucumber

1 tablespoon fresh lime juice

2 tablespoons agave syrup

¼ teaspoon sea salt

1 teaspoon apple cider vinegar

2 tablespoons filtered water

FILLING

¼ cup minced shallot

1 tablespoon chopped scallions

BATTER

1⅔ cups corn kernels (from about 3 to 4 ears of corn)

⅓ cup golden flax meal

1 tablespoon extra-virgin olive oil

1 teaspoon ground coriander

1 teaspoon minced garlic

½ teaspoon grated ginger

¼ teaspoon sea salt

¼ teaspoon freshly ground black pepper

¾ cup filtered water

Begin by placing all dipping sauce ingredients into a small bowl. Toss to mix well. Set aside to marinate.

Into food processor, place all batter ingredients. Pulse to mix, leaving the corn kernels chunky. Add filling ingredients, pulse lightly to mix.

Scoop ¼-cup portions onto a lined dehydrator tray. Dehydrate 5 to 6 hours at 104°F. Flip over and pull away the liner. Dry another 5 to 6 hours to desired consistency.

Serve with dipping sauce. Fritters keep for a week or more when fully dried. Sauce will keep for 3 days in fridge.

DOSAS WITH VEGETABLES AND DIPPING SAUCES

India

MAKES 4 SERVINGS

A *dosa* is an Indian crepe, somewhat like a thin pancake that's traditionally made using rice and lentil flour, then served with chutneys. My recipe uses coconut, and the dosa is rolled up with filling inside.

Coconut meat will range from more gelatinous and wet in texture to drier and harder. So, depending on your coconuts, you may or may not need to add additional water when blending your wrapper. Just add enough water to blend into a smooth thick cream.

 If you don't have a dehydrator yet, you can use your oven on the lowest setting to dry your wrappers on a baking tray. To keep it as raw as possible, prop open your oven door with a chopstick. This method is hardly eco green, but I'm hoping you may be inspired to acquire a dehydrator. Or, if you're craving something cooked, try using spelt or brown rice tortillas as your wrappers.

WRAPPER
1 batch Coconut Wrappers, page 178, or
    Pineapple Coconut Wrappers, page 179
1 teaspoon curry powder

FILLING
1 batch of Yellow Coconut Curry Vegetables,
    page 150, or
1 batch of Kreamed Curry Saag Spinach, page 111

DIPPING SAUCE
1 batch Tamarind Sauce, page 166, and/or
1 batch Tomato Dal, page 169, and/or
1 batch Tomato Mango Sambal, page 229

To make your wrappers, follow instructions for Coconut Wrappers, page 178. Instead of circles, place wrappers on flat surface and cut each into four squares.

To assemble dosas, place each wrapper square onto a flat surface. Scoop on about ⅓ to ½ cup filling at bottom edge. Roll filling up inside wrapper. Place on serving dish. Serve immediately with sides of dipping sauces.

Wrappers will keep for a couple of weeks in your fridge. I usually just roll them up in the ParaFlexx (the reusable nonstick dehydrator liners) and put them in a plastic bag. Or, you can store in airtight container stacked with pieces of plastic wrap or parchment paper between wrappers to keep them from sticking to one another.

COCONUT WRAPPERS

India

FILLS TWO 14-INCH EXCALIBUR DEHYDRATOR TRAYS

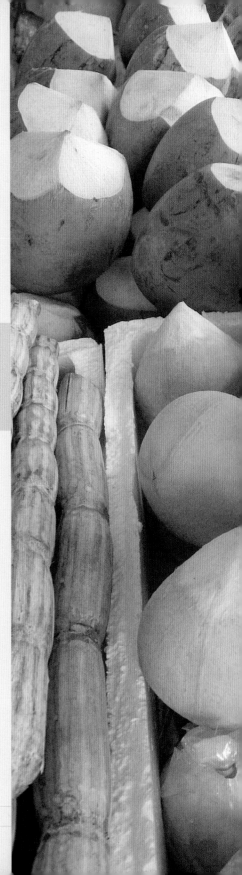

These wrappers are made by blending coconut meat from Thai baby coconuts with the least amount of water needed to make a thick cream texture. A pinch of sea salt is added for flavor. Use these wrappers cut in a square to roll up your favorite fillings, cut in a circle to enjoy with Moo Shoo Vegetables (page 180), or as the base for your savory Asian vegetable pancakes.

4 cups Thai young coconut meat, from about 5 Thai baby coconuts

½ teaspoon sea salt

1 cup coconut water, as needed

To make your Coconut Wrapper, place coconut meat in blender with salt. Blend smooth, adding only enough water, if at all, to create a thick cream texture.

Spread batter evenly onto two lined 14-inch Excalibur dehydrator trays. Dehydrate at 104°F for 4 to 6 hours, until completely dry. Remove wrappers from dehydrator, and peel away the ParaFlexx sheet carefully. Place wrapper on flat surface.

To cut into circles, use a bowl as a stencil, and cut into a total of four circles per tray. Or, cut into four squares per tray.

Wrappers will keep for a couple of weeks in your fridge. I usually just roll them up in the ParaFlexx and put them in a plastic bag. Or, you can store in an airtight container stacked with pieces of plastic wrap or parchment paper between wrappers to keep them from sticking to one another.

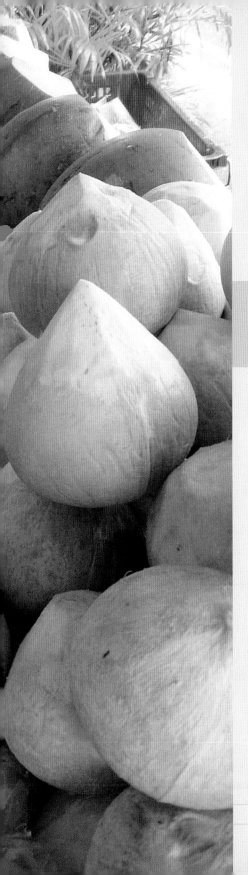

PINEAPPLE COCONUT WRAPPERS

Vietnam

FILLS TWO 14-INCH EXCALIBUR DEHYDRATOR TRAYS

This is a sweet variation of Coconut Wrappers, made by blending in pineapple for a sweeter twist that works great with savory curries and sauces. In Indonesia, the villa I stayed in would serve pancakes with chunks for pineapple for breakfast. That's what inspired this recipe.

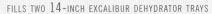

4 cups Thai young coconut meat, from about 5 Thai baby coconuts

1¼ cup diced pineapple, as needed

To make your Pineapple Coconut Wrapper, place coconut meat in blender with pineapple. Blend smooth to create a thick cream texture. Add a tablespoon of water at a time if you need more liquid to keep the mix going in the blender.

Spread batter evenly onto two lined 14-inch Excalibur dehydrator trays. Dehydrate at 104°F for 4 to 6 hours, until completely dry. Remove wrappers from dehydrator, and peel away the ParaFlexx sheet carefully. Place wrapper on flat surface.

To cut into circles, use a bowl as a stencil, and cut into a total of four circles per tray. Or, cut into four squares per tray.

Wrappers will keep for a couple weeks in your fridge. I usually just roll them up in the ParaFlexx and put them in a plastic bag. Or, you can store in airtight container stacked with pieces of plastic wrap or parchment paper between wrappers to keep them from sticking to one another.

MOO SHOO VEGETABLES WITH HOISIN SAUCE

China

MAKES 4 SERVINGS

Moo Shoo is a Chinese crepe stuffed with sautéed cabbage and mushrooms. I remember eating these for the first time in New York City's Chinatown and loving the chewy wrappers and cooked cabbage with saltiness of hoisin.

If you don't have a dehydrator yet, you can use your oven on the lowest setting to dry your wrappers on a baking tray. To keep it as raw as possible, prop open your oven door with a chopstick. This method is hardly eco green, but I'm hoping you may be inspired to acquire a dehydrator. Or, if you're craving something cooked, try using spelt or brown rice tortillas as your wrappers.

HOISIN SAUCE (CHINESE)

4 tablespoons Nama Shoyu

¼ cup raw almond butter

¼ cup yacon syrup, or 1 tablespoon agave syrup

4 teaspoons toasted sesame oil

¼ teaspoon minced garlic

Dash of black pepper, to taste

WRAPPER

1 batch Coconut Wrappers, page 178,
    cut into circles.

FILLING

1 cup sliced mushrooms, wood ear or shiitake

4 cups thinly sliced green cabbage

½ cup sliced scallion, diagonally cut into
    2-inch lengths

MARINADE

2 tablespoons toasted sesame oil

1 tablespoon extra-virgin olive oil

½ tablespoon grated ginger

1 teaspoon minced garlic

To make your sauce, place Hoisin Sauce ingredients into a small bowl and whisk together until mixed well. Set aside.

Place filling ingredients into a large mixing bowl. Add marinade ingredients and toss to mix well. Set aside for 20 minutes or longer to marinate and soften. Add ¼ cup Hoisin Sauce and toss well before serving.

To serve, transfer filling into one family style serving dish or four individual plates. Serve with a side of Coconut Wrappers and remaining Hoisin Sauce.

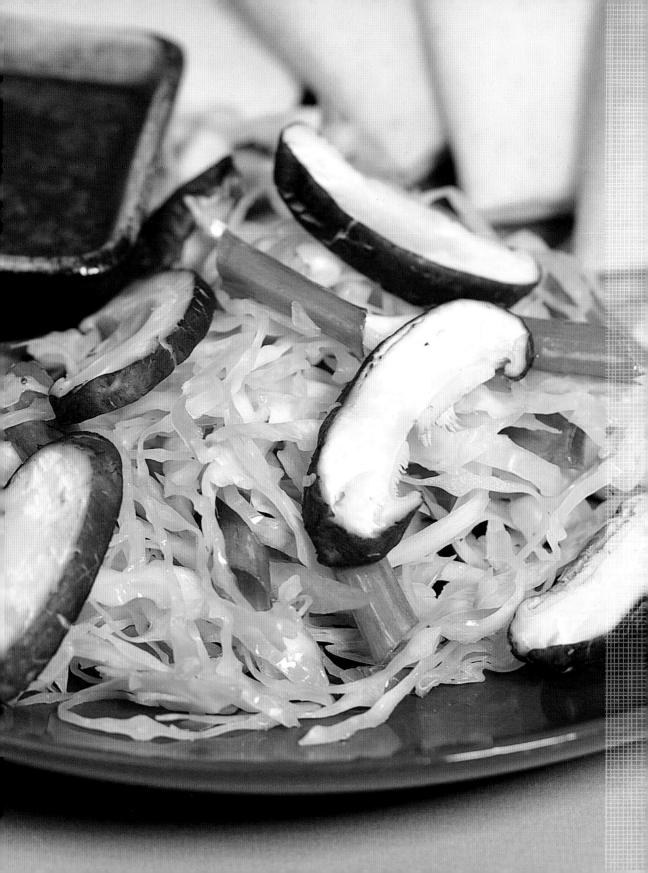

SCALLION PANCAKES WITH SPICY SESAME OIL DIPPING SAUCE

Korea

MAKES 4 SERVINGS

Pajun is Korean for scallion pancakes. It's enjoyed as a snack, appetizer, or side dish. I make the batter with coconut meat, then fill it with scallions, then dehydrate it for a few hours. It's served with a traditional Korean sesame dipping sauce made with chile, unpasteurized soy sauce, and apple cider vinegar.

If you don't have a dehydrator yet, you can use your oven on the lowest setting to dry your pancakes on a baking tray. To keep it as raw as possible, prop open your oven door with a chopstick. This method is hardly eco green, but I'm hoping you may be inspired to acquire a dehydrator.

FILLING
1 cup sliced scallions, cut into 3-inch diagonals

½ teaspoon sea salt

Dash black pepper

BATTER
1 batch Coconut Wrappers, page 178

SPICY SESAME OIL DIPPING SAUCE
¼ cup Nama Shoyu

3 tablespoons apple cider vinegar

1 tablespoon toasted sesame oil

1 tablespoon red chile flakes

1 tablespoon thinly sliced scallions

1 teaspoon minced garlic

Toss scallions with salt and pepper. Set aside.

Scoop coconut wrapper batter into center of two lined 14-inch dehydrator trays, spreading batter into an even layer about ¼ inch thick, shaped in a large circle using the back of a spoon. Evenly layer scallions over batter, and lightly press down, very gently.

Dehydrate at 104°F for 4 to 6 hours, until completely dry.

To make dipping sauce, place all ingredients into a bowl and whisk together.

To serve, cut each circle into four to six wedges. Serve with dipping sauce.

Pajun will keep for 5 days or longer in fridge. Dipping sauce will keep for a week in fridge.

VARIATIONS: *Try using other vegetables like julienned carrots, zucchini, mushrooms, and/or sliced kimchi.*

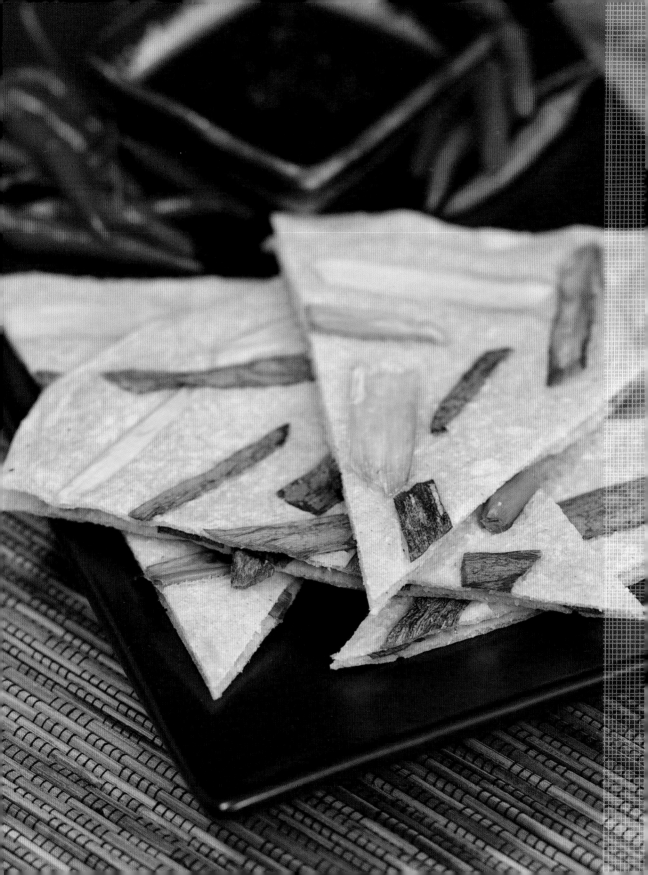

SPRING ROLLS WITH MANGO DIPPING SAUCE

Indonesia

MAKES 4 SERVINGS

Lumpia Goreng is a deep-fried Indonesian-style spring roll that's filled with bamboo and/or water chestnuts, carrots, and onion, seasoned with a garlic and shallot paste. Since bamboo doesn't taste good raw, I'm substituting with zucchini instead. Vegetables are wrapped in a Coconut Wrapper, then dehydrated.

FILLING

1 cup julienned zucchini (about 1 medium zucchini)

1 cup shredded green cabbage

½ cup julienned carrots (about 1 small carrot)

½ cup mung bean sprouts

3 tablespoons thinly sliced scallion

2 tablespoons extra-virgin olive oil

WRAPPER

1 batch Coconut Wrappers, page 178, or Pineapple Coconut Wrappers, page 179, cut into 8 squares (4 squares per tray).

PASTE

1 teaspoon minced garlic

½ cup sliced shallot

¼ teaspoon pepper

¼ teaspoon sea salt

DIPPING SAUCE

1 batch Mango Dipping Sauce, see page 185

Place filling ingredients into a mixing bowl. Toss to mix well. Set aside to soften for at least 20 minutes.

Finely pound paste ingredients in a mortar and pestle. Add to filling, and toss to mix together well.

To assemble spring rolls, scoop about ⅓ cup filling into the center of a wrapper square. Roll up, tucking in the edges to contain filling.

Serve immediately with a side of Mango Dipping Sauce.

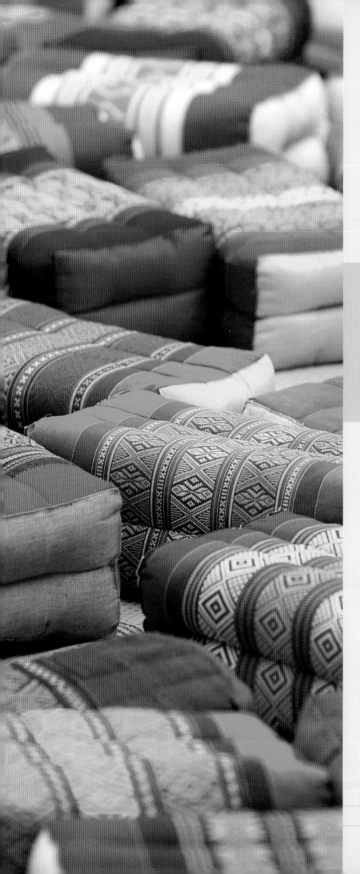

MANGO DIPPING SAUCE

Vietnam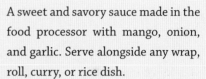

MAKES ABOUT 2 CUPS

A sweet and savory sauce made in the food processor with mango, onion, and garlic. Serve alongside any wrap, roll, curry, or rice dish.

2 cups diced mango

2 tablespoons chopped yellow onion

1 teaspoon minced garlic

¼ teaspoon sea salt

⅛ teaspoon white pepper

2 teaspoons agave syrup

Place all sauce ingredients into a food processor. Pulse lightly to mix, being careful not to over-process. You want to maintain a chunky texture.

MUSHROOM "BUL GO GI"

Korea

MAKES 4 SERVINGS

Bul Go Gi is all about the sweet and salty marinade. The beef recipe is popular in the West and is typically barbequed at the table in restaurants. Bul Go Gi is served with a stack of red leaf lettuce used to wrap namuls and kimchi. This wrap is called *sam* in Korean.

Many people have requested a raw vegan "Bul Go Gi" recipe, so I've created this version for them. I substitute beef with mushrooms marinated with the same traditional flavors.

My recipe calls for Asian pear, but you can use any ripe pear instead.

Use marinated Mushroom "Bul Go Gi" in lettuce or daikon wraps, on top of noodles and salads, in nori rolls, on its own, and as an accompaniment to any dish.

MARINADE

3 tablespoons Nama Shoyu or tamari

2 tablespoons agave, maple, or brown rice syrup, to taste

1 tablespoon toasted sesame oil

½ tablespoon minced garlic

½ cup Asian pear, microplaned or pureed in food processor, from about ½ medium pear

MUSHROOMS

4 cups sliced shiitake, miyake, oyster, or portabella mushrooms

Whisk marinade together in mixing bowl. Then, add mushrooms and massage with hands to mix well. Set aside to marinate for about 20 to 30 minutes, until softened. Squeeze liquid from mushrooms before using.

MUSHROOM "BUL GO GI"—FILLED DAIKON WRAPS

Korea

MAKES 4 SERVINGS

Sweet and salty marinated mushrooms are wrapped in thin slices of daikon rounds with marinated vegetables called namuls and pickled vegetables like kimchi. The daikon wrapper is a modern trend in South Korea today.

WRAPS
8 daikon rounds sliced as thinly as possible using a mandoline slicer
2 teaspoons agave or brown rice syrup
1 teaspoon apple cider vinegar

BUL GO GI
1 batch Mushroom "Bul Go Gi," page 186

FILLINGS
Your favorite namuls and kimchis

To prepare your wraps, place daikon, syrup, and vinegar into a mixing bowl. Mix well, and set aside for 20 to 30 minutes, until softened.

To serve, squeeze liquid from mushrooms, and place onto a serving dish. Add daikon rounds to the serving dish. Serve with your favorite marinated namul vegetables and kimchi(s) so everyone can wrap their own daikon rounds with "Bul Go Gi" mushrooms.

Best enjoyed immediately. Will keep for 2 to 3 days when mushrooms are stored separately from wraps in fridge.

MUSHROOM "BUL GO GI" LETTUCE WRAPS

Korea

MAKES 4 SERVINGS

This is a traditional style of *sam*, a Korean lettuce wrap recipe. The lettuce and Gochujang sauce are what tie this dish together. The lettuce wraps are filled with sliced garlic and pepper for savory flavors that pair with the sweet and salty marinade of the Mushroom "Bul Go Gi." Cucumber and carrot add color and texture. Try filling with your favorite marinated vegetable namuls, too, pages 94–104.

FILLINGS

1 batch Gochujang, page 225

1 clove thinly sliced garlic

1 Korean pepper, or jalapeño, sliced

1 cup julienned cucumber

1 cup julienned carrot

BUL GO GI

1 batch Mushroom "Bul Go Gi," page 186

WRAPPERS

8 red lettuce leaves, or more

To serve, place fillings and Mushroom "Bul Go Gi" into individual bowls. Place lettuce leaves in a stack on a plate.

Allow everyone to make individual wraps by placing a lettuce in their hand and stuffing with Gochujang, fillings, and Mushroom "Bul Go Gi." Wrap and eat immediately.

Will keep for several days in fridge when all ingredients are stored separately.

"RICE" WITH CATSUP AND VEGETABLES IN COCONUT WRAPPERS

Korea

MAKES 4 SERVINGS

A popular late-night dish served at coffee shops and bars after a night of dancing and drinking in Seoul, South Korea. Traditionally, rice is stir-fried with vegetables and catsup, and then stuffed inside a circle of scrambled egg that's folded in half, like an omelet. This dish is called *Om-Rice* in Korea, and is served with catsup, just like an American omelet. My version uses a square Coconut Wrapper that holds it all together.

This Sundried Tomato Catsup recipe is from *Ani's Raw Food Kitchen*, page 129.

CATSUP

1½ cups diced tomato

3 tablespoons pitted dates

¼ cup extra-virgin olive oil

1 teaspoon sea salt

1 tablespoon apple cider vinegar

½ cup sun-dried tomatoes

WRAPPER

1 batch Coconut Wrappers, page 178, cut into
    4 rectangles (cut each dehydrator tray in
    half to form 2 rectangles)

VEGETABLE RICE

1 batch Cashew Nut "Rice," page 221

½ cup diced red bell pepper

½ cup corn kernels

¼ cup diced carrots

¼ cup chopped yellow onion

1 teaspoon minced garlic, from about 1 clove

To make catsup, blend tomato, dates, oil, salt, and vinegar smooth. Add sun-dried tomatoes last and blend until thick and mixed well. Set aside.

To make vegetable rice, place all ingredients in a mixing bowl and toss to mix well. Add ¼ cup Sun-Dried Tomato Catsup, as desired, and mix well.

To serve, lay each Coconut Wrapper rectangle on one of four plates. Scoop vegetable rice onto one half of wrapper. Fold wrapper over the top of the rice. Drizzle with catsup, and serve immediately.

Best enjoyed immediately once assembled. Store rice separately from wrappers. Rice will keep 2 to 3 days when stored separately. Catsup will keep for 4 to 5 days in fridge stored on its own.

SUMMER ROLLS WITH A MUSTARD SOY SAUCE AND A KIWI SAUCE

Vietnam

MAKES 4 SERVINGS

Inspired by Vietnamese spring rolls, these rolls are filled with strips of julienned carrot, bell peppers, and cucumbers, plus mushrooms, bean sprouts, cilantro, Thai basil, and a red lettuce leaf, all rolled up inside a Coconut Wrapper. Serve with two sauces: a sweet Mustard Soy Sauce and a fresh Kiwi Sauce.

MUSTARD SOY SAUCE

¼ cup diced pineapple

1 tablespoon agave, brown rice, or maple syrup

2 tablespoons apple cider vinegar

2 tablespoons lemon juice, about 1 large lemon

2 tablespoons Nama Shoyu or tamari

1 teaspoon mustard powder, to taste

½ teaspoon minced garlic

KIWI SAUCE

¼ cup diced pineapple

½ cup peeled, diced kiwi, from 2 whole kiwi

3 tablespoons extra-virgin olive oil

1½ tablespoons apple cider vinegar

1½ tablespoons agave, brown rice,
    or maple syrup

2 tablespoons white onion

½ teaspoon sea salt

WRAPPER

1 batch Coconut Wrappers, page 178, or
    Pineapple Coconut Wrappers, page 179,
    cut into a total of 8 squares (4 per tray)

FILLINGS

8 small red lettuce leaves

1 cup julienned carrot, from 1 carrot

1 cup julienned red bell pepper, from 1 pepper

1 cup sliced mushrooms, any type

1 cup julienned cucumbers, from 1 whole

1 cup bean sprouts

¼ cup cilantro

¼ cup Thai basil, or regular basil

KIMCHI WRAPS

Korea

MAKES 4 SERVINGS

To make Mustard Soy Sauce, place ingredients into a food processor. Process to mix evenly. Scoop into a bowl, and set aside.

To make Kiwi Sauce, place ingredients into a food processor. Process to mix evenly. Set aside.

To make rolls, place wrapper square onto a flat surface. Lay down a lettuce leaf onto wrapper, then top with carrot, pepper, mushrooms, cucumbers, sprouts, cilantro, and basil. Roll up fillings inside wrapper.

To serve, place rolls onto a serving dish and serve with both sauces.

SERVING SUGGESTION: *Serve with Almond Butter Sauce, page 117.*

I learned about this innovative wrap from my cousin Minnie, who helped me perfect it, raw-style. Though Minnie's Korean, she's lived in countries all over the world including England, Saudi Arabia, Canada, and the United States. Along her journeys, she's always gravitated to a traditional Korean diet and makes really delicious kimchis. Now that she has children, she and I both came to appreciate how much our healthy, whole, fresh, and raw food diets come from our Korean heritage and culture. It was how we were raised, and I can see it in the way she feeds her children today.

FILLING
¼ cup chopped chives or scallions

1½ cups enoki mushrooms

½ cup julienned cucumber

1 tablespoon toasted sesame oil

1 tablespoon agave, brown rice, or maple syrup

WRAPPERS
8 strips of White Kimchi, page 88, or Easy Kimchi,
    page 87, in strips, rinsed slightly in filtered water
    to remove some of the spice

Place filling ingredients into a mixing bowl and use your hands to massage and mix well.

Lay a kimchi wrapper on a flat surface. Add fillings, roll up, and serve.

Best enjoyed immediately, but will keep for a day or 2 in fridge.

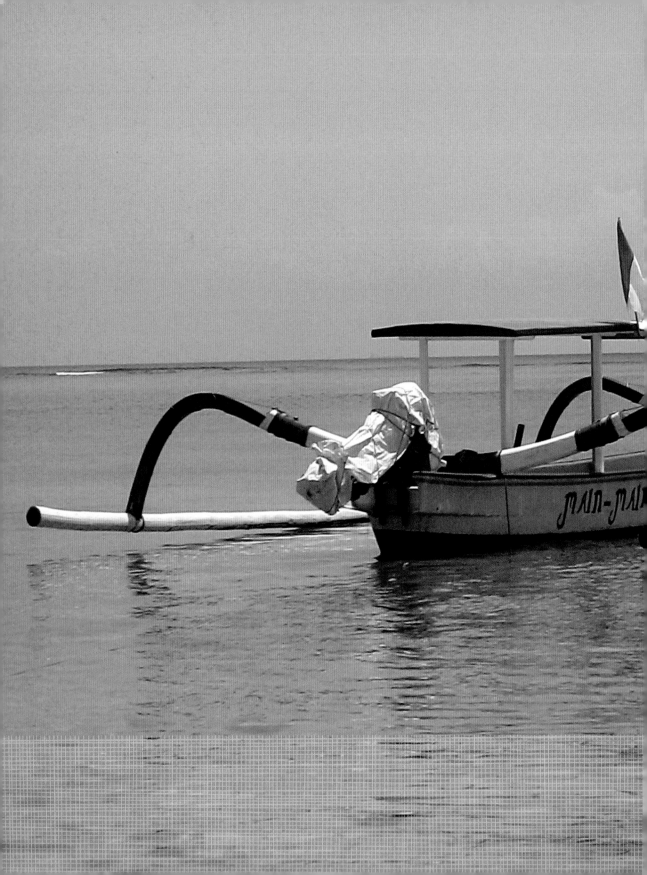

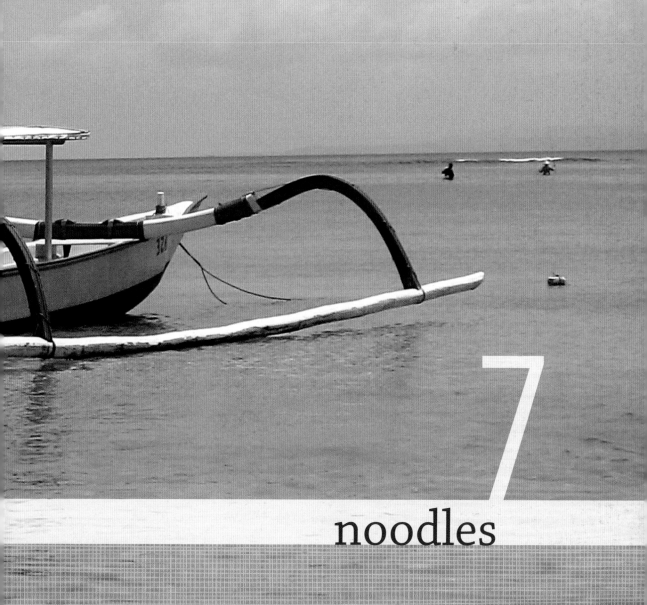

7

noodles

Rest and Recovery

Rest and recovery is an important aspect of living a long, healthy, super life. Whether it's after a stressful day or a challenging workout, this is when our body repairs and rebuilds itself to make us healthier and stronger.

When we exercise our muscles break down. The more we exercise, the greater the degradation of muscle. After any workout, muscles need to replace elements, protein, and energy stores. When we don't give our muscles enough time to recover, they become progressively smaller. This means less muscle mass, which slows down our metabolism. This is counterproductive to losing weight.

To help muscles recover, make sure to eat adequate calories (for me, that's at least 1,600 calories a day, though I usually eat more), eat some protein at every meal, get plenty of sleep, and rest at least a day between hard workouts.

When training for competition, the marathon runner and tri-athlete's immune system is lowered because overall stress levels are increased. Even they will schedule in a day of rest each week to compensate and restore.

Foods that help us recover and regenerate include sea vegetables like chlorella and spirulina, maca, hemp protein, wheatgrass, and antioxidant-rich fruits and vegetables.

PLAY

Try gentle stretching exercises or cross-train with lower-intensity activities between formal workout days. Think of it as play, just like when we used to play outside as kids, have fun, and be happy. Vary the intensity of your workouts during the week, mix up the types of exercises within your program to avoid injury and to keep your body challenged, and take at least one day off a week to rest.

SLEEP

Rest and sleep are critical to weight loss and increased metabolism. Without it, cortisol levels increase and estrogen levels in women decrease, causing weight gain around the midsection. Sleep is when our body revitalizes and rejuvenates itself to build new healthy cells that help us live a long life.

Sleep is necessary for everyone, and especially the serious athlete. Establish sleep habits and go to bed at the same time daily and try to get eight hours or more of sleep to peak your fitness levels.

I used to reach for caffeine from tea and cacao when I felt tired. Today, I'd rather feel when I am tired so I know that my body needs me to rest. We get sick when we stop listening to our body, when we fail to give it rest when it's tired. It's our body's way of forcing us to take some down-time. I haven't had a cold or flu for over a decade because of my diet, and also because I've learned to listen to my body better.

As much as I love to sleep, I've had my share of insomnia. Without sleep, my patience wears thin, I'm more sensitive and feel less productive and less powerful when I'm not well rested. Some tips from the Mayo Clinic for combating insomnia that have helped me include the following.

STICKING TO A SLEEP SCHEDULE
Keep the same bedtime and wake time from day to day, including weekends.

GET OUT OF BED WHEN NOT SLEEPING
If you can't sleep, get out of bed after 15 minutes and do something relaxing, such as reading.

AVOID TRYING TO SLEEP
The harder we try, the more awake we become. Read or watch television, if you have one, until you become very drowsy, then go to bed to sleep.

USE YOUR BED AND BEDROOM ONLY FOR SLEEPING OR INTIMATE RELATIONS
Don't read, watch TV, work, or eat in bed.

FIND WAYS TO RELAX
Take a warm bath before bedtime, ask your partner to give you a massage, create a relaxing bedtime ritual like reading, soft music, breathing exercises, yoga, or prayer. I like to meditate before bed.

AVOID OR LIMIT NAPS
Naps make it harder to fall asleep at night. If you have to take a nap, limit it to no more than 30 minutes, and don't nap after 3 p.m.

MAKE YOUR BEDROOM COMFORTABLE FOR SLEEP
Keep your bedroom dark and close your bedroom door or create a subtle background noise, such as a running fan, to help drown out other noises. Don't keep a computer, cell phone, or TV in your bedroom.

EXERCISE AND STAY ACTIVE
Get at least 20 to 30 minutes of exercise daily at least five to six hours before bedtime.

AVOID OR LIMIT CAFFEINE, ALCOHOL, AND NICOTINE

Caffeine after lunchtime and using nicotine can keep you from falling asleep at night. Alcohol, while it may initially make you feel sleepy, can cause unrestful sleep and frequent awakenings.

AVOID LARGE MEALS AND BEVERAGES BEFORE BED

A light snack is fine, but eating too much late in the evening can interfere with sleep. Drink less before bedtime so that you won't have to go to the toilet as often.

HIDE THE BEDROOM CLOCKS

Set your alarm so that you know when to get up, but then hide all clocks in your bedroom. The less you know what time it is at night, the better you'll sleep.

Noodles

The first written account of noodles dates back to between A.D. 25 and 220 in China. The oldest noodles have been discovered in Qinghai, China, and were made from millet. Today, Chinese noodles are usually made from rice flour, mung bean starch, and wheat flour.

Popular Japanese noodles are ramen, a thin wheat flour noodle; soba, a thicker noodle made from buckwheat flour; and udon, which is the thickest of the Japanese noodles, made with wheat flour. In China noodles are made Szechwan style, braised or stir-fried with pungent garlic and spicy chile peppers, while in Japan noodles are typically served in a clear broth with mild spices.

In Korea, long noodles are eaten on your birthday as a symbol for living a long life. Korean noodle dishes are served in either a hot or cold clear broth or massaged with sauce and vegetables and served cold. In Japan and Korea, slurping loudly when eating noodles is customary and considered to be a compliment to the chef.

KELP NOODLES

The raw noodles I love to use in place of the cooked buckwheat, wheat, or mung bean noodles are kelp noodles. Kelp is a sea vegetable full of minerals from the ocean, vitamins, iodine, and other healthy nutrients. The noodles have only about 6 calories a serving, and have a mild flavor that carries the flavors of whatever sauce or broth they're served with. The colder the noodles are, the crunchier they become, making them a great addition to salads. And, the warmer the noodles are, the softer the texture is. Leaving kelp noodles to soak up marinade in a bowl for 30 minutes or longer softens them even further.

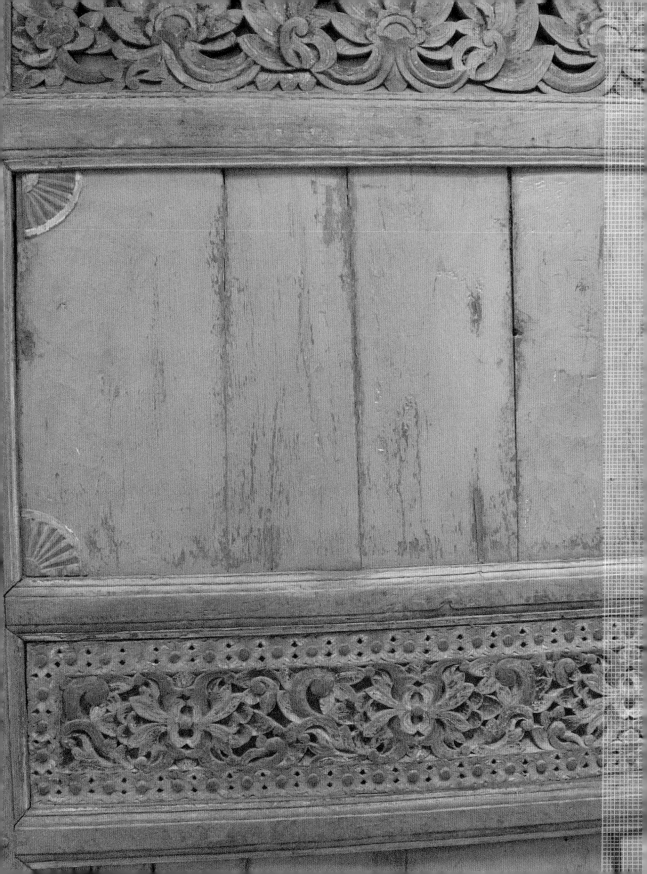

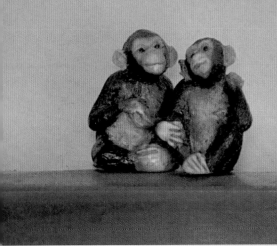

Sea vegetables are an age-old Asian secret for longevity and beauty (see page 140) and they're known as the ultimate super food. Kelp noodles boost our immune system, make us healthier, and help us live a long super life.

Kelp noodles are easy to find at most health food stores and Korean or Asian markets. They're also available online at www.GoSuperLife.com. If you can't find kelp noodles, you can simply substitute with your favorite vegetable noodles.

VEGETABLE NOODLES

Noodles can be made by using a spiral slicer (available at www.GoSuperLife.com) to cut vegetables like zucchini or carrots into long, thin strands similar in shape to angel hair pasta.

Use vegetable noodles in the same way you would any noodle, and feel free to substitute kelp noodles if you can't find them.

COCONUT NOODLES

The meat from a Thai baby coconut can be sliced into long strands to make coconut noodles.

Use coconut noodles alone, or mixed with vegetable noodles in place of or in addition to kelp noodles in the following recipes.

 If you're craving cooked noodles, feel free to substitute any of my raw kelp, vegetable, or coconut noodles with a buckwheat (soba) or rice noodle. Note that some buckwheat noodles mix buckwheat with wheat flour, so make sure to read the ingredients if you have a gluten allergy. And, if you're wanting something warm or hot, heat up my recipes in a saucepan to your desired temperature. I like to dip my finger in the pot to make sure it doesn't get too warm since I like to keep my temperatures below 104°F for the biggest nutritional pop.

SUKIYAKI MUSHROOMS WITH NOODLES

Japan

MAKES 4 SERVINGS

Sukiyaki is a popular one-pot meal in Japan that's simmered in a skillet or pan in a sauce with vegetables and tofu or meat. It's usually cooked at the table and it's common to eat with others from the same pan, which makes it a fun party dish for sharing.

The clear broth is easy to make by hydrating wakame, then soy sauce–flavored marinated mushrooms, bok choy, Chinese cabbage, carrots, and kelp noodles are added in.

BROTH
⅓ cup dried wakame
4 cups filtered water
3 tablespoons agave syrup

VEGETABLES
1 cup sliced mixed mushrooms, like enoki, miyake, and shiitake
1 cup thinly sliced baby bok choy
1 cup thinly sliced Chinese cabbage
½ cup julienned carrot
¼ cup Nama Shoyu

NOODLES
4 cups kelp noodles (about 1 pound of noodles)

Place wakame, water, and agave syrup into mixing bowl. Set aside 30 minutes to hydrate.

Place all vegetable ingredients into mixing bowl. Toss to mix well. Set aside 30 minutes or longer to marinate and soften.

To serve, portion broth into four serving bowls. Add noodles. Top with vegetables and marinade.

Broth will keep for 4 days when stored separately in fridge. Marinated vegetables will keep 1 day stored separately in fridge. Assembled noodles will keep 1 day in fridge.

SPICY MIXED VEGETABLE NOODLES

Korea

MAKES 4 SERVINGS

This dish is called *Bibim Gooksoo* in Korean. The word *bibim* means "mixed," and *gooksoo* are "noodles." This Korean spicy mixed-noodle recipe is traditionally served cold and made with buckwheat noodles. I substitute with nutritious, low-calorie kelp noodles and give it my California twist by adding in romaine for greens.

In Korea, noodles are enjoyed on a birthday to symbolize a long life. Last year my Korean girlfriend took me out for noodles to celebrate my birthday, and the noodles I ate inspired my recipe for Spicy Mixed Vegetable Noodles.

SAUCE

1 batch Gochujang, page 225

1 tablespoon Nama Shoyu

1 tablespoon apple cider vinegar

½ teaspoon minced garlic

NOODLES

4 cups kelp noodles (about 1 pound of noodles), rinsed, drained

TOPPINGS

1 cup cored, peeled, thinly sliced Asian or bosc pear (about 1 pear)

1 cup julienned cucumber (about 1 cucumber)

2 cups sliced romaine leaves

½ cup Daikon Kimchi, page 91, or Easy Kimchi, page 87, optional

Whisk together sauce ingredients in a mixing bowl.

Add noodles to sauce, toss to mix well. Add toppings and mix well.

To serve, transfer to four bowls, and enjoy immediately.

GLASS NOODLES WITH MARINATED MUSHROOMS, SPINACH, AND CARROTS

Korea

MAKES 4 SERVINGS

A Korean dish traditionally made with sweet potato noodles. In this recipe, vegetables are marinated in soy, toasted sesame oil, and minced garlic and then tossed with kelp noodles. Meaty mushrooms, orange carrots, green spinach, and onion make this a festive and colorful dish.

MARINADE

2 tablespoons Nama Shoyu

2 tablespoons toasted sesame oil

2 tablespoons agave syrup

¾ teaspoon minced garlic

VEGETABLES

1 cup thinly sliced shiitake or wood ear mushroom

¼ cup thinly sliced yellow onion

1 cup julienned carrots (about 1 carrot)

NOODLES

4 cups kelp noodles (about 1 pound of noodles)

2 cups washed, dried, and lightly packed spinach

3 tablespoons sliced scallion, cut into 1-inch lengths

GARNISH

2 tablespoons sesame seeds

In a mixing bowl, whisk together marinade ingredients. Add vegetables to marinade. Toss to mix. Set aside to marinate and soften for at least 20 minutes.

Add noodles, spinach, and scallion to bowl with marinated vegetables. Toss to mix well.

To serve, transfer to a serving dish or four bowls. Top with sesame seeds and enjoy immediately.

This dish is best eaten immediately, but will keep for 1 day in fridge.

"FRIED" VEGETABLE NOODLES WITH "DEEP-FRIED" SHALLOTS

Indonesia

MAKES 4 SERVINGS

I first tasted pan-fried egg noodles called *Bakmi Goreng* on a visit to tropical Bali when it was served for breakfast at the resort I was staying at, and the dish reminded me of a vegetable stir-fried Chinese noodle recipe.

I later found out my host was of Chinese decent, and her family had been living in Jakarta for many, many generations. Unlike Korea, Indonesian culture is a beautiful mix of influences and people from different Asian countries, including India and China.

MARINADE

3 tablespoons extra-virgin olive oil

2 tablespoons Nama Shoyu

1 teaspoon minced garlic

¼ teaspoon white pepper, to taste

NOODLES

4 cups kelp noodles (about 1 pound of noodles)

GARNISH

1 batch "Deep-Fried" Shallots, page 206

VEGETABLES

1 cup shredded baby bok choy leaves,
   or green cabbage

½ cup julienned carrots (about ½ carrot)

½ cup crumbled cauliflower

¼ cup thinly sliced shallots

3 tablespoons sliced scallions, cut in
   1-inch lengths

Whisk marinade ingredients in mixing bowl. Add vegetables, and toss to mix well. Set aside for at least 20 minutes to marinate and soften.

Add kelp noodles to bowl with marinade and vegetables, toss and mix well. Serve immediately, or set aside another hour for the noodles to marinate and soften.

To serve, transfer to four serving dishes. Sprinkle with "Deep-Fried" Shallots just before serving.

This dish is best eaten immediately, but tossed noodles will keep for 1 day in fridge.

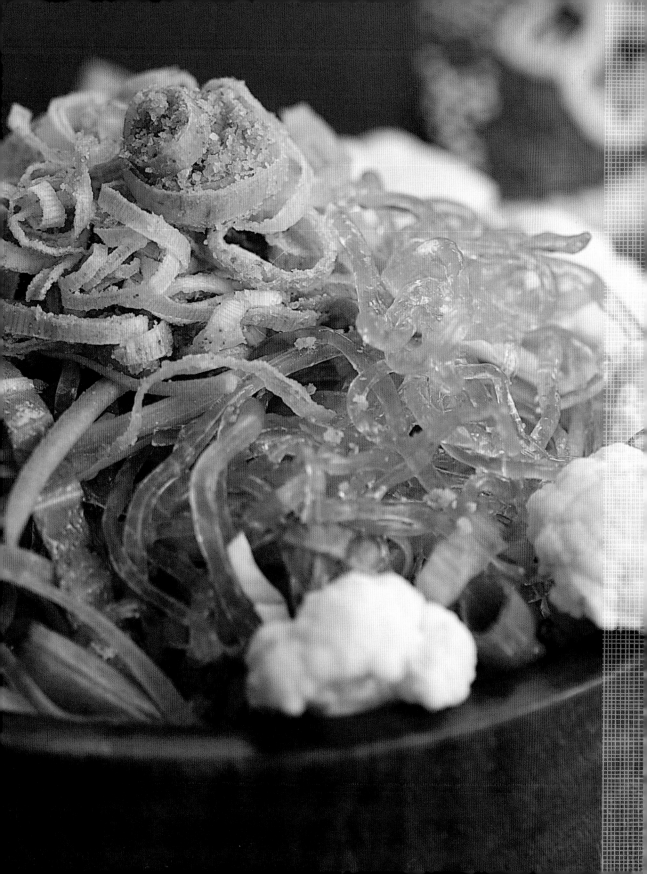

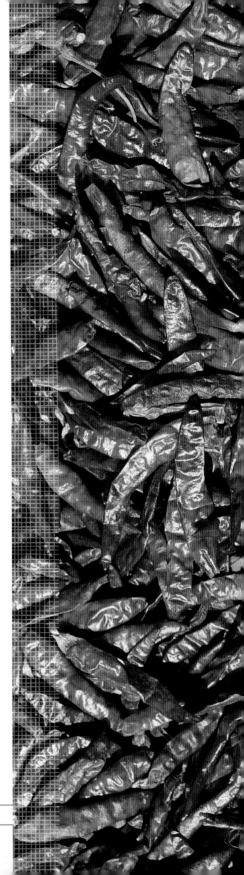

HEALTHY ASIAN CUISINE

In traditional Asian diets, plant-based food makes up the core daily intake, including rice, grains, fruit, and vegetables (including sea vegetables), nuts, seeds, herbs, spices, and plant-based drinks like tea, wine, and beer. Eating this way provides all essential micronutrients like vitamins and minerals, fiber, and other plant substances that promote health. Minimal processing and the freshness of foods also maximize their fiber, antioxidant, and nutritional values.

Asian diets are characteristically low in saturated and total fat, and are absent, except in India, of dairy products. As a matter of fact, most Asians are lactose-intolerant. The plant-based, dairy-free diets of Asia are associated with low incidence of osteoporosis, diabetes, heart disease, and obesity. Some may think Asian women are at higher risks for osteoporosis, but that's due to their thinner and smaller-boned frame, not their diet. Weight-bearing and regular exercise like walking, jogging, dancing, and weight training, along with a healthy, well-balanced diet rich in calcium (from leafy green vegetables and many nuts) and vitamin D help combat osteoporosis.

In China, Taoism influences the belief in food as a way to a long life. Food is deemed medicinal, and is classified according to medicinal properties. For example, ginger heats the blood and is good for people with anemia. Balancing of the condition of the body is sought through food. In Japan, traditionally Buddhists don't believe in killing, so they won't eat meat or fish.

Evidence increasingly shows us consumption of meat, especially red meats, increases chronic diseases like heart disease and cancer. Meat doesn't have dietary fiber or antioxidant nutrients and is only used as a seasoning in traditional Asian cuisine, if at all.

>>>

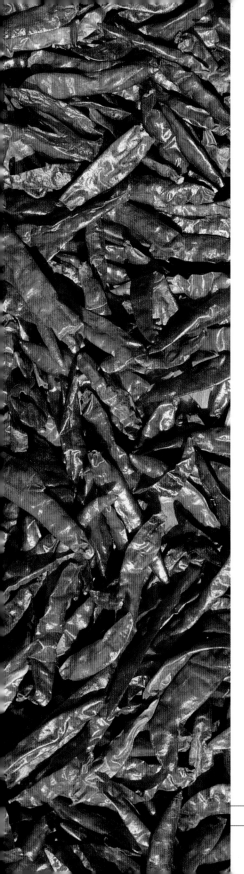

Black and green teas are sipped all day long and are full of antioxidants contributing to the low rates of chronic diseases.

Regular physical activity that links mind, body, and spirit, and other lifestyle factors, like the social support and pleasure of sharing food with family and friends, also contribute to the high life expectancy and low chronic disease rates found in most of Asia.

Here are some healthy ingredients common in Asian cuisine:

- Cilantro, basil, mint, garlic, and other herbs and spices contain antibacterial compounds as well as cholesterol-lowering properties, dietary fiber, and magnesium.

- Red chile is good for the blood and cardiovascular system. The capsaicin in chile switches on metabolism to help people burn fat and lose weight and is the active ingredient found in most natural weight-loss pills.

- Turmeric is a ginger-like spice critical in Indian curry; it contains curcumin, which is thought to fight cancer and Alzheimer's disease. It's also a strong anti-inflammatory agent, and is high in iron and manganese.

- Raw and fermented foods are common, and if cooked, they are only cooked lightly in a small amount of oil. Fermented foods are full of friendly bacteria that build stronger digestion, aid in absorption of nutrients, and elimination of waste from our body. Probiotics in fermented foods boost our immune system and make us stronger.

"DEEP-FRIED" SHALLOTS

Japan

MAKES 4 SERVINGS

 This recipe is inspired by my popular Buckwheat Battered "Fried" Onion Rings from *Ani's Raw Food Essentials*. Thinly sliced shallots are tossed in a light batter of buckwheat flour, then dehydrated until crispy. "Deep-Fried" Shallots add a light crispy crunch and are a great topping for wraps, sandwiches, soups, salads, and noodles.

BATTER

2 cups buckwheat groats, ground into a powder

1 teaspoon sea salt

½ teaspoon cayenne powder

SHALLOTS

4 cups thinly sliced shallots

3 tablespoons extra-virgin olive oil

2 tablespoons filtered water

Toss together batter ingredients, set aside.

Into mixing bowl, place shallot ingredients. Toss to mix well. Dip shallots into batter to coat well.

Place shallots in single layer onto two lined 14-inch Excalibur dehydrator trays. Dry at 104°F for 4 to 6 hours, until dry and crisp.

If you don't have a dehydrator, you can dry these in your oven at the lowest temperature. You could prop the oven door open with a spoon or butter knife, but that's hardly eco. Hopefully you'll love the outcome and be inspired to acquire a dehydrator for your kitchen.

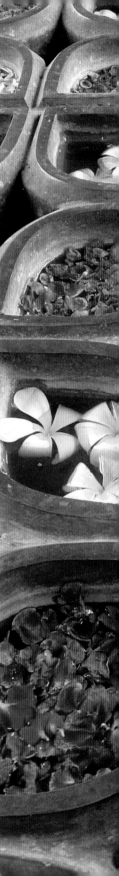

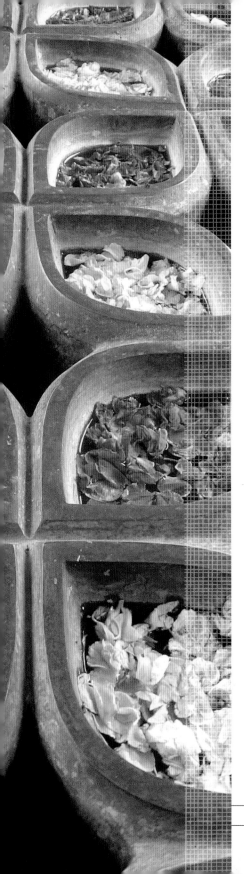

BUCKWHEAT GROATS

Groats means a hulled seed. Yes, buckwheat is a seed, not a wheat, so it's gluten-free. They're a great lower-fat source of protein than nuts. Ideally, I like to soak buckwheat groats in triple the amount of filtered water overnight, then rinse them to thoroughly remove gooeyness. The groats grow and expand when soaked.

I then spread a thin layer of soaked groats onto a lined dehydrator tray and dry them at 104°F for 3 to 5 hours, until completely dry. I call these my Buckwheat Crispies, and keep them on hand in a glass jar for months. Enjoy with a nut mylk as a morning cereal, top salads and add to rolls and wraps for added crunch, or grind into a powder to coat vegetables, as in my "Deep-Fried" Shallots recipe, page 206.

Buckwheat groats are one of the easiest seeds to sprout. To sprout about 1 cup, follow these directions:

Place ⅔ cup buckwheat groats into a bowl. Add 2 cups filtered water. Set aside to soak for 30 minutes. Do not over-soak groats and don't soak longer than 1 hour, or they will not sprout.

Empty seeds into sprouter and drain off soak water. Rinse well with fresh water until the water runs clear and is no longer thick and gooey. Drain well.

Rinse and drain again in 4 to 8 hours. Then, set out of direct sunlight at room temperature. Repeat two or three more times, until you see small tails growing. Sprouts are ready to eat 8 to 12 hours after final rinse. Drain fully before storing.

Store spouts in glass container or plastic bag in fridge. Enjoy quickly, as they will continue to grow slowly in your fridge.

NOODLES AND VEGETABLES IN A RED CURRY SAUCE
Thailand

MAKES 4 SERVINGS

Gueyteow Pak is the Thai dish inspiring this recipe. Bean sprouts, string beans, and coconut milk are tossed in a red curry paste known as *Nam Prik Gaeng Ped*. Then, kelp noodles are added in and garnished with almonds, cilantro, and lime wedges.

CURRY SAUCE

1 cup Coconut Milk, page 144

1 tablespoon Red Curry Paste, page 209

¾ teaspoon curry powder

2 teaspoons agave or maple syrup

VEGETABLES

1 cup mung bean sprouts

1 cup sliced string beans, cut into
    1-inch lengths

½ cup stemmed, julienned broccoli

3 tablespoons finely sliced shallot

NOODLES

4 cups kelp noodles (about 1 pound of noodles)

GARNISH

3 tablespoons crushed almonds

2 tablespoons chopped cilantro

4 lime wedges

Combine all curry sauce ingredients in a mixing bowl. Add noodles and set aside for 1 hour to marinate and soften.

Add vegetables to sauce and noodles. Toss to mix well.

To serve, portion noodles and sauce into four bowls. Top with almonds, cilantro, and lime wedges.

Curry sauce will keep for 3 days in fridge when stored separately. The noodles are best eaten immediately, but tossed noodles will keep for 1 day in fridge.

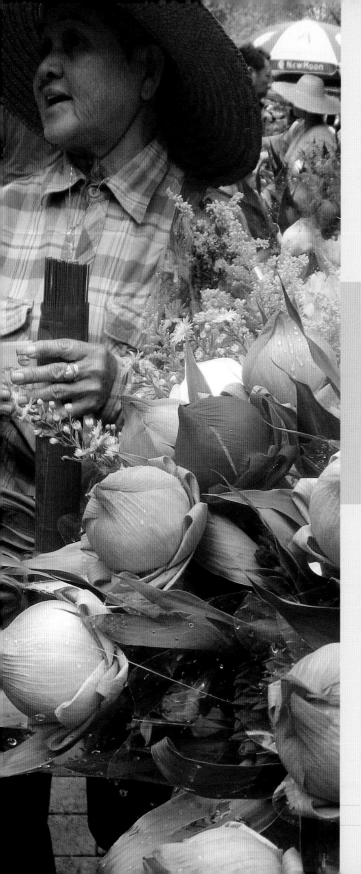

RED CURRY PASTE
Thailand

MAKES ABOUT 3 TABLESPOONS

Nam Prik Gaeng Ped is Thai red curry paste, which is the base for most Thai curries. This paste is concentrated and fragrant. Mix with coconut milk to make a red curry sauce.

2 tablespoons chopped yellow onion

1 tablespoon chopped lemongrass

1 teaspoon minced garlic

½ teaspoon grated ginger

¼ to ½ teaspoon cayenne powder, to taste

¼ teaspoon ground cumin

⅛ teaspoon sea salt

½ tablespoon extra-virgin olive oil

In mortar and pestle, mix onion, lemongrass, garlic, ginger, cayenne, cumin, and salt into paste. Add oil and mix together well.

Will keep for 5 days in fridge.

NOODLES IN SEAWEED BROTH WITH JAPANESE SEVEN-SPICE

Japan

MAKES 4 SERVINGS

This broth's flavor comes from the sea vegetables dulse and/or wakame and shiitake mushrooms. Noodles are added and topped with sesame seeds, scallion, and a Seven-Spice Seasoning, then garnished with beautiful Lotus Root Chips.

BROTH

4 cups filtered water

⅓ cup dried dulse, and/or wakame

¼ cup Nama Shoyu, to taste

3 tablespoons apple cider vinegar

2 tablespoons agave syrup

NOODLES

4 cups noodles from either a 1-pound package
    of kelp noodles, and/or 2 cups coconut
    meat, and/or 2 cups zucchini noodles

GARNISH

2 teaspoons sesame seeds

2 tablespoons sliced scallion

½ batch Lotus Root Chips, page 124

1 batch Japanese Seven-Spice Seasoning,
    page 211

Combine broth ingredients in a blender. Before blending, set aside 30 minutes to hydrate. Then, blend smooth. Pour broth through strainer into bowl.

If using kelp noodles, rinse well. If using coconut meat, open coconut (see Opening a Coconut, page 27). Use the back side of a spoon to scrape out the coconut meat and slice into thin noodles. If using zucchini, either spiralize them or slice them thinly lengthwise, and then into long thin strips. You want to have a total of 4 cups of noodles.

To serve, scoop soup broth into four serving bowls. Add 1 cup of noodles. Garnish with sesame seeds, scallion, and Lotus Root Chips. Serve with a side of Seven-Spice Seasoning.

Broth will keep for 5 days in fridge when stored separately.

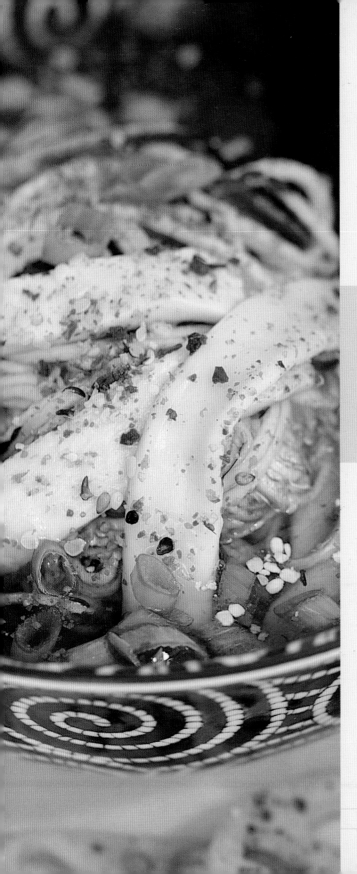

SEVEN-SPICE SEASONING

Japan

MAKES ¼ CUP

Shichimi Togarashi, or Japanese seven-spice seasoning is commonly found at Japanese restaurants. This seasoning is great on soups, salads, wraps, and noodles to add heat and color.

2 teaspoons cayenne powder

2 teaspoons crushed hemp seed

2 teaspoons crushed sesame seed

2 teaspoons grated dried
      orange peel

2 teaspoons dried nori flakes

2 teaspoons ginger powder

Grind and mix together all ingredients.

Will keep for months stored in airtight container in fridge.

VEGETARIAN PHO WITH VEGETABLES AND HOISIN SAUCE

Vietnam

MAKES 4 SERVINGS

Many Vietnamese people eat *pho* for breakfast rather than as an evening meal. The broth for this recipe is made by blending ginger, garlic, and bay leaf and then adding in marinated onion and mushrooms. Kelp noodles are placed in the broth along with basil, cilantro, scallions, and greens. Serve with a side of bean sprouts and Hoisin Sauce.

MARINADE

¼ cup diced yellow onion

½ cup sliced button mushrooms

¼ cup Nama Shoyu or Bragg Liquid Aminos

BROTH

1 tablespoon grated ginger

1 teaspoon minced garlic

1 bay leaf

4 cups filtered water

NOODLES

4 cups kelp noodles (about 1 pound of noodles)

VEGETABLES

½ cup shredded napa cabbage

½ cup tender greens like mustard, Bibb, red leaf, mache, or spinach

⅓ cup basil leaves

⅓ cup coarsely chopped fresh cilantro

2 tablespoons thinly sliced scallions

GARNISH

1 cup bean sprouts

1 lime, cut into wedges

1 fresh red or green chile pepper, sliced

1 batch Hoisin Sauce, page 213

Marinate onion and mushrooms by tossing in a bowl with Nama Shoyu. Set aside for 20 minutes to marinate and soften.

Make broth by placing ginger, garlic, bay leaf, and 1 cup water in blender. Blend smooth. Add remaining water and the onion marinade mixture. Pulse lightly to mix.

Place noodles into four serving bowls. Put vegetables on top of noodles in each bowl. Pour broth into each bowl.

Place vegetable garnish onto one plate. Serve as a side along with Hoisin Sauce.

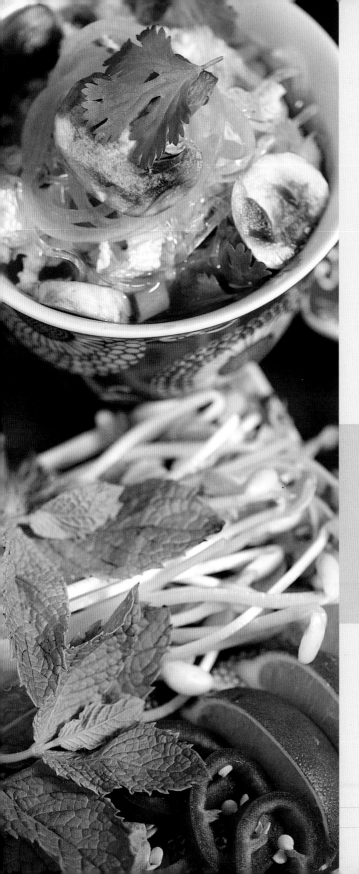

HOISIN SAUCE

Vietnam

MAKES ½ CUP

Hoisin sauce is typically a Chinese dipping sauce traditionally made with sugar, soybeans, vinegar, salt, garlic, chile. This is my Vietnamese-inspired version to enjoy with your Pho. To add a rich flavor, I like to use yacon syrup, which is lower in sugar and calories than agave syrup and has the flavor of molasses. If you don't have yacon syrup, you can use agave syrup, brown rice syrup, or honey (which is not considered vegan) instead.

¼ cup Nama Shoyu

2 tablespoons almond butter

2 to 3 tablespoons yacon syrup, to taste

2 teaspoons apple cider vinegar

2 teaspoons toasted sesame oil

½ teaspoon minced garlic

Pinch cayenne powder, to taste

Place all ingredients into a small bowl. Whisk until mixed well.

Will keep a week or longer in the fridge.

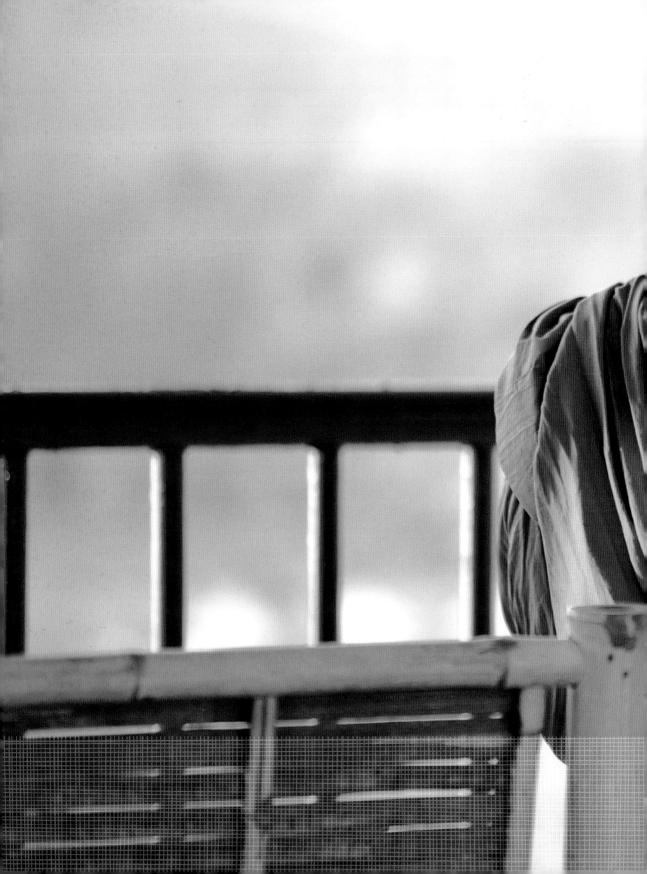

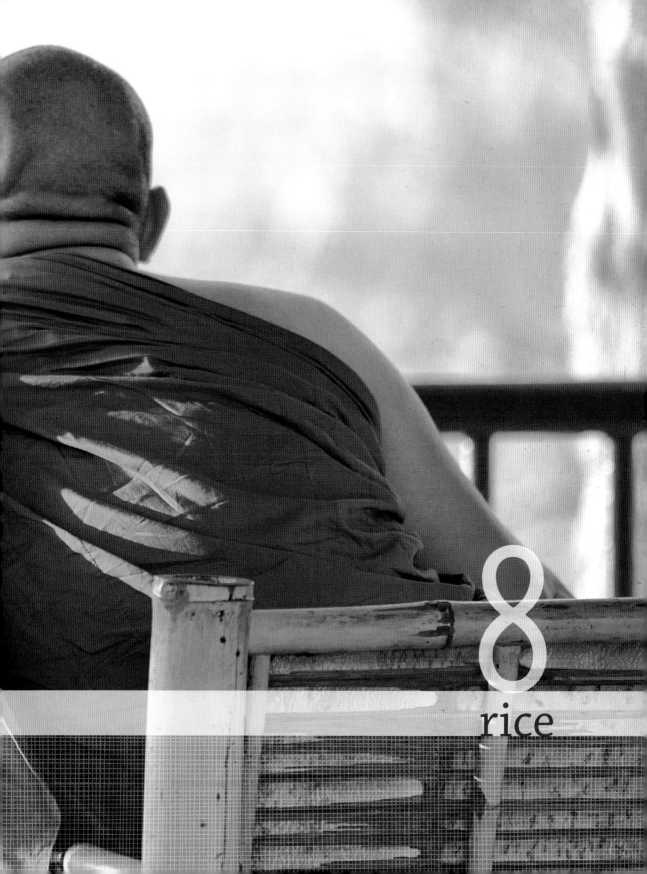

8
rice

Social Fitness

Beyond nutrition, clean and toxin-free living, physical fitness, and rest, how we interact with one another affects our mental and spiritual health and, in turn, our longevity.

Acting with dignity, respect, and honor for myself and for others, instead of from a place of fear, lack, and desperation, helps me make better decisions while avoiding hurting myself and others. Spending time with inspiring people whom I look up to as positive role models and who help me to grow is one way to keep on my game.

There are always cultural differences to take into account when interacting with people. One big difference in communication styles in Korea vs. the United States is that here in the States we feel it's polite to make conversation by asking questions to engage another person. Especially to an older Korean person, it's seen as disrespectful to lead the conversation by aggressively asking questions. I remember being told to speak only when addressed and to only answer questions when asked by an elder. Too much chatter is seen as poor etiquette. While most of my friends' dinner tables here in the United States were where family gathered to share news about their day, dinners in our home were always quiet and peaceful.

These are other skills I continue to practice and develop:

BE A GOOD LISTENER

Being a good listener reflects our level of social fitness. When someone's speaking, it helps me to count to thirty in my head before saying anything. I'm usually eager to jump in to give my 2 cents or response, but waiting 30 seconds helps me give the other person enough time to finish their thought. Sometimes, it feels uncomfortable to sit silently, waiting. But what I've found to happen is that just when I thought the other person said it all, he or she will continue to reach deeper down to share even more. Easier said than done, but I also try to listen neutrally, without getting emotionally defensive.

CLEAR COMMUNICATION

Communication is a two-way street. Just because I've said something won't always mean the message was clearly received on the other end. Try asking the other person to repeat back to you what they think you said. You may be surprised that your message wasn't as clearly received as you'd thought. After someone has told me something, I like to rephrase what he or she said to confirm I've heard the message loud and clear.

In Asian cultures, one doesn't want to draw attention to oneself. Everything is about the good for the group, rather than an individual. And, when an elder says something, it's never questioned or challenged, even when you disagree. I found this to be very frustrating.

TOLERANCE AND ACCEPTANCE

I celebrate the fact that our world is a beautifully rich patchwork made up of many different cultures, ethnicities, and points of view. I practice keeping an open mind to see if I might learn something new from someone else's perspective. Everyone has a unique story. Discussion, sharing, learning, and growing together with others is what I believe life is about. I always felt we encounter people for a reason, whether for 5 minutes or 50 years, perhaps to have a certain experience that enriches our life.

Melding East and West cultures is about tolerance and acceptance for different beliefs and communication styles. There are always positives and negatives everywhere; appreciating the best of both places is something I continue to work on in my life.

EMOTIONAL MATURITY

Controlling our emotions instead of letting them get the better of us is emotional maturity. People who are emotionally mature take accountability for their life and actions. They have patience, genuinely care for others, act honestly, and keep self-control and balance in all things. Emotionally mature people can talk about things that may be upsetting and share feelings and emotions appropriately.

This is the most challenging piece I continue to work on daily by working hard to achieve my goals, accepting and working through tensions and worries, and learning to bear pain, hurt, and life's uncertainties. Life is not always a bed of flowers. I try my best to face consequences for things I've done, like hurting someone's feelings, and learn from my mistakes. I accept my failures, see them as opportunities to learn and grow, and make better decisions moving forward. Through the ups and downs, I strive to keep a positive approach and to always do my best to make time to help others.

The one piece I have the most challenge with is recognizing and expressing my anger. The stereotype of the Asian woman is one that is more passive, submissive, quiet, and sweet. In Eastern religions and ways of thought, things are usually accepted as they are. We push things off onto karma to make right in the next lifetime for us.

It's important for me to work on releasing my anger, even if it means punching pillows in a closed room or screaming in my car on the freeway. It still feels strange when I do it, but it's supposed to be good for me in the long run.

BE HAPPY

Feeling happy adds to our level of mental fitness. When we feel confident and good about ourselves, we won't have time to gossip because we're instead busy focusing on what we want. We will be too busy creating good and positive change in the world around us that will hopefully help make someone else's life even better.

AVOID TV

I haven't had a television for about twenty years and haven't watched much of it in my life. These days, it's easy to watch episodes online, and I'll watch interesting documentaries, and on occasion, an episode or two of a show that doesn't seem to hold my attention for long. Most of the programming on TV is designed to be dramatic, fast paced, exciting, and in many ways unhealthy.

Food shows, I love the concept of them. But the hosts typically use ingredients I avoid, like white flour, butter, sugar, animal products, and processed and packaged foods. A majority of the hosts are overweight, don't look healthy, and they don't reflect a balanced, active lifestyle, nor longevity. I strive to build a lean, strong, radiant, healthy body. So, I can't look to a chef using unhealthy ingredients to show me how to make food. Eat their food, and I'll look like them. No thank you.

After returning to the States from my first trip to southeast Asia, where I stayed for 6 weeks, I began to notice our diverse, multicultural reality here in the United States is not represented on our American TV. A very narrow subsection of our culture is portrayed in a way that I can't relate to. A world of drama, lying, cheating, and hurting one another. People watch what's on TV and use what they see to define their reality of social fitness. We're all connected, and it's vital to treat each other with dignity, respect, and honor to avoid drama, not create it.

RESPECT AND HONOR

A person's honor is his integrity and doing right in all situations. Respect can mean being polite, but I use it to mean treating other people better than ourselves. Asian culture puts the good of the community over the good of one individual. Education is held in high regard, as is wisdom that can only come with age. A friend once said "Let's treat one another as prophets, instead of for profit."

Let's all take on more accountability by understanding the impact of our actions. Let's be committed to being respectful, to honor all living beings, and to fight for justice. In Asia we have many ceremonies honoring our ancestors and those who have come before us. These are the giants whose shoulders we stand upon, and it's important to remember to give credit where credit is due. We wouldn't have the opportunities we have had someone before us not created them for us.

BE A SPIRITUAL WARRIOR

Awareness, courage, and gentleness are the traits of a spiritual warrior. I love that combination!

There's a saying on the island of Lombok in Indonesia: "It's nice to be important, but more important to be nice." In Lombok, people purposefully choose to smile and be happy.

Rice

Rice is Asia's staple food—3.7 billion Asians live on rice—and central to the Asian way of life, culture, customs, traditions, and spirituality. It's a backbreaking chore to plant rice; every seedling must be poked into the mud by hand. My grandfather had numerous rice fields in the countryside of southern South Korea where he was famous for his rice wine brew called *makali*. I used to love visiting as a child, seeing the expanse of green rice patty fields was beautiful.

I make my raw version of rice using a vegetable chopped into small bits in a food processor. I prefer using vegetables light in color like turnip, daikon, or jicama. I sometimes mix in small bits of cashews or pine nuts to add a softer mouth feel. Other vegetables that work for making rice include autumn squash, cauliflower florets, and broccoli florets.

Raw, vegetable-based rice is easy to make in your food processor and can be seasoned and served the same way as cooked rice.

 If you're craving a warm rice, heat any of my recipes in a bowl placed in a small oven. Better yet, if you have a dehydrator, just place the bowl of rice inside for a couple of hours to heat up to your desired temperature. The temperature I prefer is 104°F for maximum nutritional benefits.

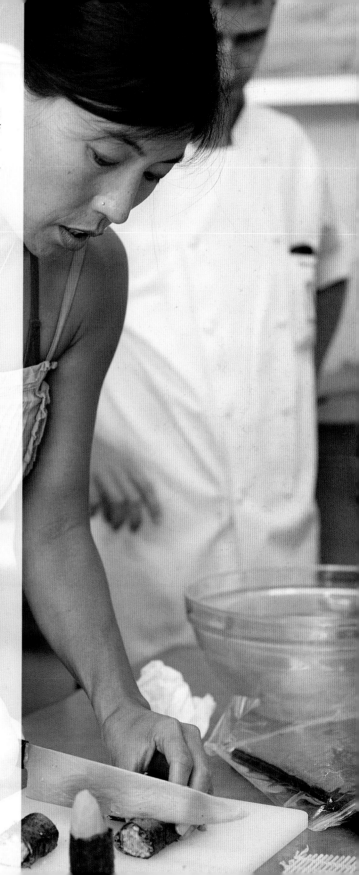

SWEET CORN "RICE" WITH LEMONGRASS CHILI

Singapore

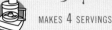

MAKES 4 SERVINGS

Nasi Jagung (sweet corn rice) is made by mixing equal parts of sweet corn with rice. It's delicious and quick to make. Serve with a tart, spicy Lemongrass Chili.

I like to eat corn to build up my glycogen stores in my body to help fuel a heavier workout. Corn is a good, starchy, complex carbohydrate. Choose organic corn to avoid genetically modified organisms and toxic pesticides and herbicides commonly used to grow corn.

LEMONGRASS CHILI

3 tablespoons finely minced lemongrass

2 tablespoons minced shallot

½ teaspoon minced garlic

½ teaspoon sea salt

½ cup extra-virgin olive oil

1 tablespoon agave or maple syrup

1 teaspoon apple cider vinegar

RICE

1 batch Cashew Nut "Rice," page 221

2 cups sweet corn kernels

1 tablespoon agave syrup, optional

In mortar and pestle, or a small food processor, grind together lemongrass, shallot, garlic, and salt. In a clean bowl, mix together with olive oil, agave syrup, and vinegar. Set aside.

In mixing bowl, toss together rice with corn and agave syrup.

To serve, transfer rice to four bowls. Serve with a side of Lemongrass Chili.

Rice will keep for 2 days in fridge. Chili will keep for 5 days in fridge.

CASHEW NUT "RICE"

Hawaii

MAKES 2 CUPS

This raw rice is made by lightly processing into small rice-size bits turnip, daikon radish, or jicama with soft cashews. I choose cashews for their color and mild flavor. Use this rice the same way you would a cooked grain rice.

Note: You want to process into small pieces. But, make sure not to over-process, or your rice will become mush.

> 1 cup cashews
> ½ teaspoon sea salt
> 3 cups peeled and diced turnips,
>   daikon radish, or jicama

In a food processor, place cashews and salt. Pulse lightly to process into small pieces. Add turnips, daikon, or jicama and pulse lightly to chop into small pieces. Be careful not to over-process into mush.

Will keep for a couple of days in fridge.

MUSHROOM "RICE"

Korea

MAKES 4 SERVINGS

Marinated mushrooms and spicy kimchi are mixed into Cashew Nut "Rice" to mimic a popular, simple Korean rice dish.

> 1 cup sliced mushrooms, any type, like shiitake,
>   straw, enokitake, oyster
> 1 teaspoon Nama Shoyu or tamari
> 1 teaspoon toasted sesame oil
> 1 batch Cashew Nut "Rice" (see left)
> ½ cup chopped kimchi
> 1 tablespoon sesame seeds, for garnish

Mix mushrooms with Nama Shoyu and sesame oil and set aside to soften and marinate for 10 minutes or longer. Squeeze excess liquid by hand before using.

Scoop rice into a mixing bowl. Add marinated mushrooms and kimchi, mix well.

To serve, scoop into serving bowl. Add sesame seeds to garnish.

Will keep for 2 days in fridge.

JICAMA "RICE" WITH SLICED SCALLIONS AND SESAME OIL

Vietnam

MAKES 2 CUPS

One of my favorite raw restaurants in California is AuLac. Situated in a neighborhood known as Little Saigon in Orange County, AuLac is where you'll find my good friend Chef Ito, along with his delicious raw menu. Many of his recipes are Asian influenced and served family style, so it's fun to meet up with a big group of friends for a meal there. Ito's delicious rice dish inspired this recipe.

Simple to make by processing jicama with miso and scallions, it's great on its own as a meal with Black and Tan Encrusted Coconut Meat (page 78) or Vegetable Tempura (page 118) added on top or as a side to any dish. Serve as you would any rice.

Note: You want to process into small pieces. But, make sure not to over-process, or your rice will become mush.

RICE

4 cups peeled, cubed jicama

1 tablespoon white miso

1 teaspoon toasted sesame oil

⅓ cup sliced scallions

TOPPING

1 batch Black and Tan Encrusted Coconut Meat, page 78 or

1 batch Vegetable Tempura, page 118

In a food processor, place jicama, miso, and sesame oil. Pulse lightly to process into small pieces, being careful not to over-process into mush. Add scallions and pulse lightly to mix, being careful not to over-process.

Will keep for a couple of days in fridge.

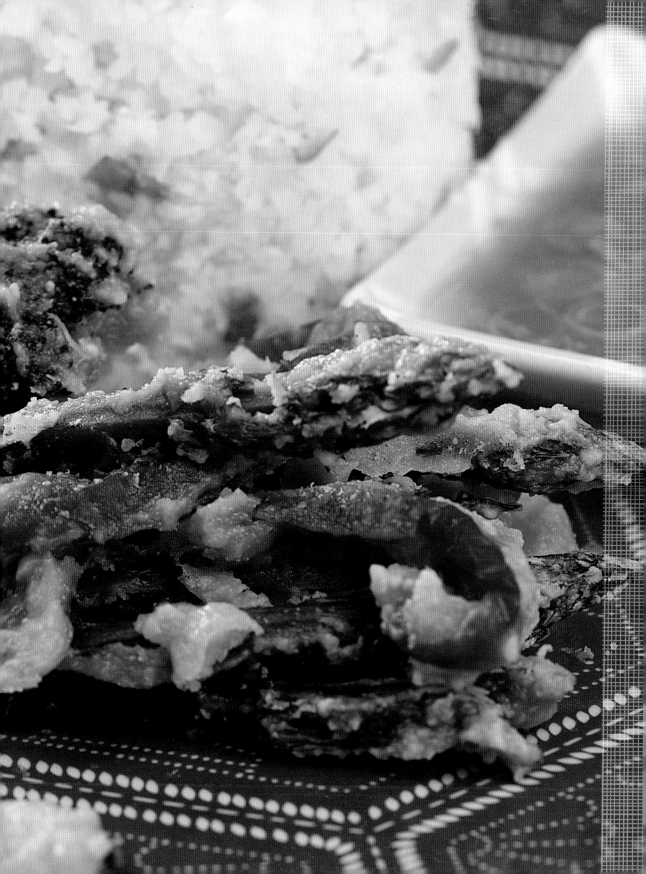

BI-BIM-BOP
(MIXED VEGETABLE "RICE")
WITH GOCHUJANG

Korea

MAKES 4 SERVINGS

Bi-bim-bop means "mixed vegetable rice." It's a popular dish in Korea where traditionally rice is placed in a large bowl, then topped with marinated vegetables and Gochujang, a hot pepper paste made of miso soybean paste, sesame, and red pepper powder. The resulting flavor is a mix of hot, sweet, salty, savory, and sour. A colorful dish with many flavors that's fun to eat.

1 batch Cashew Nut "Rice,"
    page 221

4 teaspoons toasted sesame oil

1 batch each of 4 to 6 of your
    favorite namuls, pages 94–104

1 batch Gochujang, page 225

Place rice into four serving bowls and drizzle each with 1 teaspoon sesame oil. Neatly arrange each separate namul on top of your rice. Scoop 1 to 2 teaspoons Gochujang, to taste, into center of namul.

Enjoy immediately.

Will keep for 1 to 2 days in fridge.

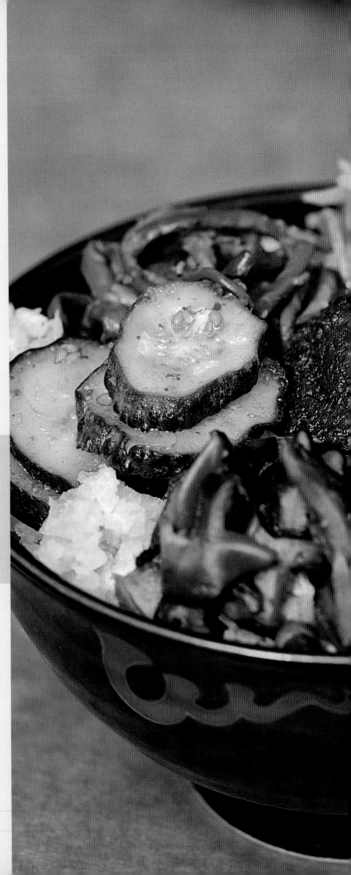

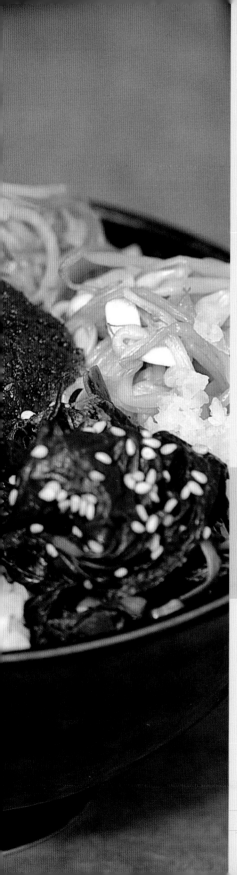

GOCHUJANG

Korea

MAKES 4 SERVINGS

Gochujang is a traditional Korean hot chile pepper paste made by adding powdered red peppers to miso soybean paste and then aging and fermenting this mixture in earthen pots outdoors under the sun. The resulting flavor is a mix of hot, sweet, salty, savory, and sour. Gochujang is the sauce used to tie together vegetables with rice to make Bi-Bim-Bop and is also used in noodle recipes and wraps. My recipe keeps for weeks in the fridge, so keep extra on hand to dress up salads and lettuce wraps and to use as a dip, too.

   If you have access to a Korean market, you can always buy real Gochujang, which usually contains sugar. Or, make your own healthier version by following this easy recipe.

2½ tablespoons unpasteurized miso, red, yellow, or brown

2 tablespoons toasted sesame oil

¼ cup agave syrup

½ teaspoon Korean chile powder, or cayenne pepper powder, to taste

Place all ingredients into a small mixing bowl, and mix well.

Will keep for several weeks in the fridge.

PINEAPPLE "FRIED RICE" WITH PINEAPPLE CURRY SAUCE

Thailand

MAKES 4 SERVINGS

Khao Phad Sapparod is the name of this Thai dish. It's made with sweet chunks of pineapple, cashews, peas, and currants and served with a Pineapple Curry Sauce.

Cut pineapple in half lengthwise and hollow out. Save the pineapple shell to serve the rice in for a festive presentation.

PINEAPPLE CURRY SAUCE

2 cups Coconut Milk, page 144

1 cup crushed fresh pineapple

2 tablespoons Red Curry Paste, page 209

1 tablespoon Nama Shoyu

1 tablespoon agave syrup

RICE

1 batch Cashew Nut "Rice," page 221

2 cups pineapple chunks

¼ cup thinly sliced shallot

½ cup peas, fresh or frozen and thawed

GARNISH

¼ cup raisins or currants

¼ cup chopped fresh cilantro

Whisk together curry sauce ingredients in a mixing bowl. Set aside.

In mixing bowl, place rice ingredients. Mix well.

To serve, transfer rice to the hollowed-out pineapple as the serving bowl or scoop it into four bowls. Ladle curry sauce over it and garnish with raisins and cilantro.

Will keep for a day in fridge.

PINEAPPLE MANGO "RICE" WITH HONEY LEMON SAUCE

Hawaii

MAKES 4 SERVINGS

A mixed rice dish inspired by a traditional Hawaiian salad that's tossed with fresh pineapple mango, raisins, walnuts, and crisp cucumber and celery. The rice is tossed in a sweet sauce made traditionally with honey, pineapple, lemon, and a touch of garlic. Honey can be substituted with your favorite sweetener like agave or brown rice syrup.

SAUCE

4 tablespoons lemon, from about 2 whole lemons

3 tablespoons honey, raw, or agave syrup, or 4 tablespoons brown rice syrup

2 tablespoons pineapple juice

½ teaspoon minced garlic, about 1 clove

Salt and pepper, to taste

RICE

1 batch Cashew Nut "Rice," page 221

¾ cup diced pineapple

½ cup diced mango

¼ cup lightly crushed walnuts

⅓ cup raisins

½ cup diced cucumber

¼ cup finely chopped celery

To make sauce, whisk together ingredients in a bowl. Set aside.

To make rice, place all ingredients into a large mixing bowl with sauce. Gently toss to mix well.

To serve, scoop into a serving dish.

Best enjoyed immediately. Will keep for a day in fridge.

COCONUT SAFFRON "RICE" WITH TOMATO MANGO SAMBAL

Indonesia

MAKES 4 SERVINGS

Coconut rice is found in Thailand and Indonesia, and it's a delicious variation on plain white rice that's made with coconut milk and shredded coconut. I love saffron, which is an expensive spice more frequently found in Indian cuisine. A little saffron goes a long way, so I use only a small amount in this recipe along with turmeric for color.

Turmeric has a long list of health benefits including the fact that it's a natural antiseptic and antibacterial agent useful in disinfecting cuts and burns; it's a natural liver detoxifier; it's been used in Chinese medicine to treat depression; and it has anti-inflammatory properties, making it useful in the treatment of arthritis.

Grinding your shredded coconut in a Personal Blender with the grinder top, or in your coffee grinder, or using a mortar and pestle will help make it easier to break it down into finer bits than when using a food processor.

RICE

1 batch Cashew Nut "Rice," page 221

¼ cup shredded coconut, ground into powder using a grinder or mortar and pestle

½ teaspoon saffron threads

½ teaspoon turmeric

¼ teaspoon minced garlic

½ teaspoon lemon juice

GARNISH

1 batch Tomato Mango Sambal, page 229

Place all rice ingredients into your food processor or a mixing bowl. Lightly pulse or toss to mix well.

Serve with a side of Tomato Mango Sambal.

TOMATO MANGO SAMBAL

Indonesia

MAKES ABOUT ¾ CUP

Sambal is a fresh, spicy, and tangy relish, sort of like a salsa in Mexican food, that's made using fruit or tomato. For less spice, remove seeds from your chiles before using.

I use mango and tomato in this recipe. You can just use either tomato or mango by using double the amount (1 cup of either).

- ½ cup chopped tomato (about ½ tomato)
- ½ cup chopped mango (about ½ mango)
- 1 tablespoon yellow onion
- 1 teaspoon fresh lime juice
- ½ teaspoon minced garlic
- ½ teaspoon chopped red chile or jalapeño, to taste
- ⅛ teaspoon sea salt

Place all ingredients into a mixing bowl. Mix well.

To serve, transfer into a serving bowl.

Will keep for two days in fridge.

GARAM MASALA

India

MAKES ABOUT 2 TABLESPOONS

This is a dry spice mixture popular in India. *Garam Masala* means "hot spice," but it's not spicy like chile peppers, but rather is aromatic and intense. It is believed to create a sense of happiness and well-being.

Garam masala mixtures vary widely across India. Common ingredients include peppercorns, clove, cumin, cinnamon, cardamom, nutmeg, star anise, and coriander. It's always best to grind your own powder from whole spices, but I'm using ground powders in this recipe for simplicity.

- 1 tablespoon cumin powder
- 1½ teaspoons cardamom powder
- 1 teaspoon ground black pepper
- 1 teaspoon ground cinnamon
- ½ teaspoon grated nutmeg
- ¼ teaspoon ground clove

Place all ingredients into a small bowl and stir to mix well.

Store in airtight container at room temperature. Will keep for several months or longer.

KASHMIRI PULAO

India

MAKES 4 SERVINGS

This is a sweeter style of rice inspired by a popular rice dish in Northern India. Spiced with cinnamon, cardamom, walnuts, and sweet raisins.

1 batch Cashew Nut "Rice," page 221

½ teaspoon cinnamon powder

½ teaspoon cardamom

½ teaspoon minced garlic

2 tablespoons lightly crushed walnuts

2 tablespoons raisins

1 tablespoon liquid coconut oil

3 rose petals, organic, for garnish

Place all ingredients, except for the rose petals, into mixing bowl. Toss to mix well.

To serve, place rice into one large bowl, or four small bowls, and garnish with finely torn rose petals.

Will keep for 2 to 3 days in fridge.

VEGETABLE PULAO

India

MAKES 4 SERVINGS

An Indian vegetable rice dish with peas, bell peppers, carrots, jalapeño, ginger, and cilantro, spiced with Garam Masala, a pungent spice mixture that offers up a flavor different from hot chile pepper spice.

1 batch Cashew Nut "Rice," page 221

1 teaspoon Garam Masala, page 229

½ cup peas, fresh or frozen and thawed

¼ cup chopped green bell pepper

¼ cup chopped carrots

½ cup chopped tomato

2 tablespoons chopped white onion

½ teaspoon chopped jalapeño, to taste

1 teaspoon minced ginger

2 tablespoons chopped cilantro leaves

1 tablespoon liquid coconut oil or
    extra-virgin olive oil

Mix rice with Garam Masala, then add in remaining ingredients. Mix well.

To serve, scoop into serving bowl.

Will keep for 3 to 4 days in fridge.

WASABI MAYO

Japan

MAKES ABOUT 1 CUP

A creamy rich mayonnaise made from blended macadamia nuts or cashews with the added kick of wasabi. Use as you would any mayonnaise, in wraps, rolls, sauces, and as a dip.

> ½ cup macadamia, cashew, or pine nuts
> ½ cup Wasabi, page 236
> ⅓ to ½ cup filtered water, as needed

Blend all ingredients into a smooth mayonnaise. Use as little water as possible to create a thick cream texture.

Will keep 4 to 5 days in fridge.

KIMCHI KIM BAP

Korea

MAKES 4 SERVINGS

A simple Korean nori roll filled with "rice" and kimchi massaged in sesame oil and sweet syrup. If you want to avoid extra calories and sugar, try using stevia powder instead. Start with a pinch, adding more gradually, as it has a strong flavor.

> 1 cup kimchi
> 1 tablespoon toasted sesame oil
> 1 tablespoon agave or brown rice syrup, or stevia powder, to taste
> 4 sheets nori paper
> 1 batch Cashew Nut "Rice," page 221

First, rinse kimchi in filtered water to remove some of the spice and salt. Drain and place into mixing bowl with sesame oil and agave syrup. Massage to mix and coat well. Place onto cutting board and chop.

To assemble your rolls, place a sheet of nori onto a flat, dry surface like a cutting board. Along the bottom third of the sheet closest to you, spread on about ⅓ cup of your rice evenly. Next, spread about ¼ cup kimchi evenly onto your rice. Roll kimchi up inside of nori, pressing lightly to bind together the fillings. The nori paper will moisten from the rice to help hold your roll together.

To serve, slice into six to eight pieces. Enjoy immediately.

WASABI MAYO, UMEBOSHI PLUM, AND SHISO LEAF NORI ROLL

Japan

MAKES 4 SERVINGS

This recipe calls for two traditional Japanese ingredients: umeboshi plum and shiso leaf.

Umeboshi plum has been used for thousands of years as a food and medicinal product. The pickled salty and tart plum stimulates metabolic activity and helps us to eliminate toxins. Look for whole umeboshi plums, but the paste will work, too. If you can't find either, substitute with sauerkraut or another pickled, tart, and salty vegetable.

Shiso leaf is the Japanese name for the perilla leaf, a perennial herb in the mint family. Perilla is also popular in Korea. It's used in Chinese medicine to stimulate the immune system, and fight colds. It tastes like a mix of basil and mint, so use those more familiar herbs if you can't find shiso.

FILLING

8 shiso leaves, or ¼ cup of mixed mint
   and basil

1 batch Wasabi Mayo, page 237

1 umeboshi plum, pitted, minced,
   or ¼ cup saurkraut

1 cup sprouts, any type

1 cup peeled, seeded, sliced avocado
   (about 1 avocado)

WRAPPER

4 nori sheets

RICE

1 batch Cashew Nut "Rice," page 221

To assemble your rolls, place a sheet of nori onto a flat, dry surface like a cutting board. Along the bottom third of the sheet closest to you, evenly layer 2 shiso leaves or 2 tablespoons of your basil and mint. Then, spread on about ⅓ cup of your rice evenly over the greens. The greens act as a moisture barrier to help keep your nori dry.

Next, spread about 2 to 3 tablespoons of Wasabi Mayo evenly onto your rice. Add about a ½ teaspoon or more, to taste, of your minced umeboshi plum or 2 tablespoons of sauerkraut. Add on about a ¼ cup of sprouts and ¼ cup avocado.

Roll fillings up inside of nori, pressing lightly to help the avocado bind together the fillings.

To serve, slice into six to eight pieces and serve with a side of pickled ginger. Enjoy immediately.

ZUCCHINI AND SHIITAKE KIM BAP WITH DAIKON

Korea

MAKES 4 SERVINGS

This is inspired by *choong moo kim bap*, a small, finger-size nori roll that's about 3 inches long and is traditionally filled with just rice and served with a sweet and tart daikon radish cut into rectangles.

My rolls are filled with spinach and shiitake namul and rice.

LONG DAIKON CUBES

2 cups diced daikon, cut into long rectangles about 2 inches long

½ teaspoon salt

½ cup apple cider vinegar

1 tablespoon Korean chile powder, or ¼ teaspoon cayenne, to taste

1 tablespoon agave or brown rice syrup or date syrup, or pinch of stevia powder

½ tablespoon Nama Shoyu or tamari

½ teaspoon minced garlic

⅛ teaspoon minced ginger

ROLLS

4 sheets nori paper

1 batch Cashew Nut "Rice," page 221

1 batch Zucchini Namul, page 98

1 batch Shiitake Mushroom Namul, page 103

First, marinate daikon cubes in salt and vinegar for 1 hour to soften. Remove from marinade and drain. Place in mixing bowl and add remaining daikon ingredients. Massage to coat and mix well. Set aside.

To assemble your rolls, place a sheet of nori onto a flat, dry surface like a cutting board. Along the bottom third of the sheet closest to you, evenly spread on about ¼ cup of your rice. Next, spread about ¼ cup of each namul evenly onto your rice.

Roll fillings up inside of nori, pressing lightly to help it bind together. The nori will get damp, helping to hold roll together.

To serve, slice into 3-inch lengths, and serve with a side of Long Daikon Cubes. Enjoy immediately.

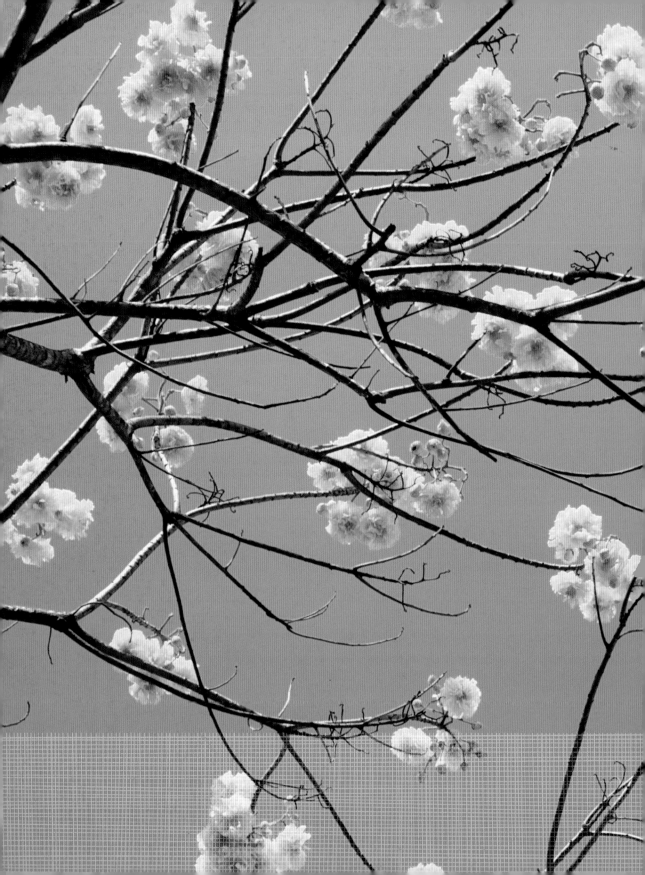

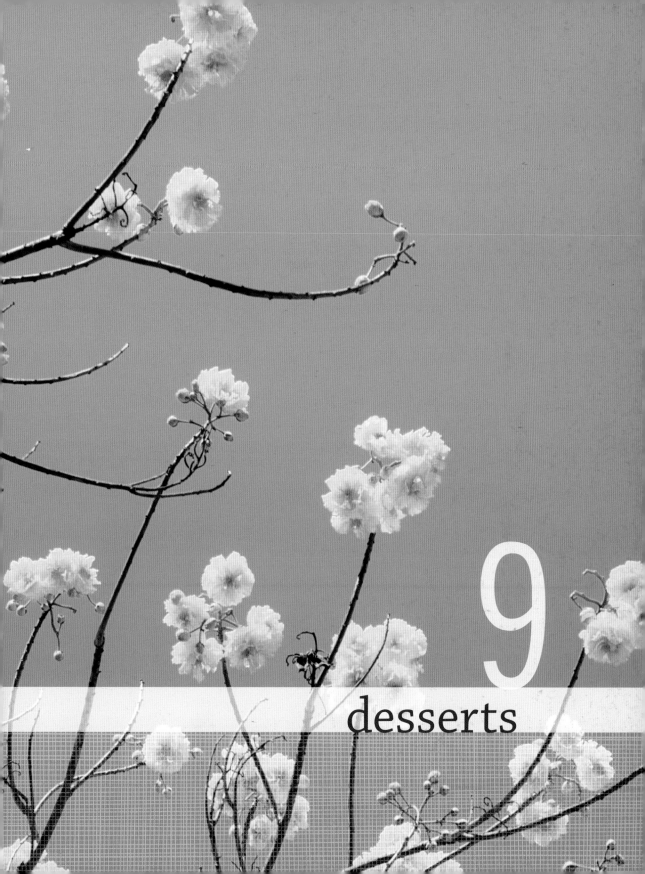

9

desserts

Happiness

The secret to lasting happiness is how we choose to behave, think, and live. Though life circumstances are often out of our control, we can choose how to deal with situations. Happy people are more flexible, resilient, and able to bounce back from adversity. When we are happier, we become more social, helpful, creative, and willing to try new things. We also become healthier and extend our life expectancy. It's about the journey, not the destination.

CHOOSE HAPPY

Choose to be happy by choosing attitudes and behaviors that will lead to happiness instead of unhappiness. Happiness is a learned behavior and a conscious decision that takes commitment and work. Proven methods for increasing happiness include developing nurturing relationships, being grateful, forgiving ourselves and others, helping others, being generous, meditating, and exercising. Each of these can become habits that become easier over time.

Dan Gilbert, Harvard psychologist, refers to a study he conducted at Harvard University and describes how we grow synthetic happiness. You can watch him speak about this on TED at http://www.ted.com/talks/dan_gilbert_asks_why_are_we_happy.html.

Two groups of students took a photography class, then took two of their favorite photos, developed and blew them up in the darkroom. At the end of the class, one group was told to choose their favorite photo to submit as evidence that they'd taken the course. This photo was mailed away. The second group was to choose their favorite photo, but was given four days in which to change their mind.

The group that was forced to make a decision and to stick to it, when surveyed days later, were found to be happier about their decision. The group that had the option to change their minds continued to wonder if they'd made the right choice and were less happy and less satisfied with their final decision.

This study demonstrated how the frontal cortex of our brain creates happiness. When we aren't given the option of choices, our brain creates happiness for us with what we are dealt. In America, we often hear the term *option paralysis*, and though we have more wealth, physical possessions, and a higher quality of life than much of the world, our happiness index is lower than that of less prosperous countries. I believe it's because we're always waiting for the next best thing to come along, rather than appreciating everything we already have.

Most spiritual practices in Asia revolve around practicing nonattachment to objects, people, circumstances, and expectations. Gratitude and giving thanks for blessings bring happiness. Prayer, focusing on good for others, helping others, and ensuring living a life of clean karma help keep the happiness index higher in Asian countries.

GRATITUDE

I've already mentioned this, and bring it in again here because an attitude of gratitude is the super highway to happiness. Counting my blessings helps me feel happier. It's as easy as thinking of ten things to be grateful for like the air I have to breathe, access to clean food and water, a healthy strong body, and loving family and friends.

In the Buddhist kingdom of Bhutan, the king claims an attitude of gratitude that fosters an environment where happiness can occur. In our Western world, it's so easy to focus on everything we don't have, rather than remembering to focus on all that we do have. It's ironic in a way, considering how much more we do have in America compared to more Third World–level countries in Asia.

FORGIVENESS

Holding onto a grudge only harms us. Research has shown grudges can affect our physical and mental health. Forgiveness is one way to let go of negative feelings.

In his book, *Five Steps to Forgiveness*, Clinical psychologist Everett Worthington recommends a five-step process he calls REACH: Recall the hurt, then Empathize to understand perpetrator's point of view, be Altruistic by remembering a time in your life when you were forgiven, Commit by writing a letter expressing forgiveness to the person or putting it into your journal, then Hold onto the forgiveness. Don't dwell on your anger or hurt because that's a form of chronic stress. Just let it all go.

FRIENDSHIP

One Australian study found people over the age of seventy with a strong network of friends lived much longer. Our increasingly individualistic society lacks meaningful social connections, which psychologists believe causes today's rise in depression. Make it a priority to nurture loving relationships.

In Asia, groups of seniors are seen gathering for meals, hikes in the mountains, tai chi or chi gong in the town square. Beyond friendship, family bonds in Asia run strong. It's customary for three or four generations to live together, and everyone helps one another. It made an impact on me to see how happy my aunt and uncle were living in a tiny two-room home with three generations and a total of nine people. I believe humans are meant to be in tribes and communities. We're not meant to live alone and to be as isolated as we've become here in the West. The mentality of good for all vs. the good of one individual helps to keep people feeling more connected in Asian countries.

GET IN THE FLOW

To be in the flow means being engaged in meaningful tasks that absorb our focus and challenge our abilities. Being in the flow makes us happy.

Research has found the most common passive, leisure-time activity of watching TV produces the lowest levels of happiness.

Our continuous bombardment by media via TV, video screens, texts, e-mails, and music keeps us entertained, but also distracts us from actively using our minds. More important, all these distractions keep us from having our own thoughts that are not influenced by what we see and hear in the media. Finding alone time to sit in quiet and to think our own thoughts is critical for our happiness.

Meditation is a common practice in many Asian countries, and schoolchildren start their day with group exercise and song giving thanks for things in their lives to help their flow kick off the day.

GENEROSITY AND HELPING OTHERS

Helping others supercharges my happiness. Getting involved in your community and volunteering for a cause you care about are great ways to improve well-being and increase longevity. These kinds of activities require interaction with people and help you to develop new skills, in turn fueling our self-esteem and self-confidence. Helping others has even been found to alleviate aches and pains in the body.

Stephen G. Post, Ph.D., co-author of *Why Good Things Happen to Good People: The Exciting New Research That Proves the Link Between Doing Good and Living a Longer, Healthier, Happier Life*, says mood elevation from helping others is associated with a release of serotonin, endorphins (the body's natural opiates), and oxytocin (a compassion hormone) that reinforces even more helping behavior. A National Academy of Sciences 2006 study showed just thinking about contributing to a charity activates the brain's reward center, which is associated with feelings of joy.

In Asian countries where the good of the group is a higher priority than the good of just one person, resources, like food, are shared. Monks carry a bowl with them, and it is filled with rice by families because Asians respect the role of the monk as praying and meditating to set good vibrations and intentions for the good of the community.

PETS

Studies have shown pets decrease stress and make us feel happiness, laughter, love, and warmth. Kanga, my Rhodesian Ridgeback, reminds me to go on long walks in nature, to stop and smell the roses, lie in the sun, and take naps. She gives me perspective and reminds me whatever seems to be so important at the moment, really isn't.

Pets are a modern occurrence in Asia. And many times, pets live outside the house. It's different than here in the West, where pets are your family.

HAPPINESS ECONOMICS

Happiness economics is an interesting field of study in which a country's quality of life is calculated by combining economics with psychology. Studies have found money correlates with levels of happiness, but the rate diminishes as money increases. Things that do increase happiness include the amount of spare time we have, the level of control we have over our spare time, and feeling in control of our life.

As the amount of money we have increases, happiness has been found to decrease because we are too focused on acquiring things and being consumers. We adapt quickly to changes like a new job, car, or house, which is why acquiring things may boost happiness for a second, but fades quickly. We need to keep upping the ante to boost our happiness again and again. It's important to realize we are not consumers, but people.

Native tribes worked only three hours daily to secure food and shelter. Today, we work eight to twelve hour days. To put this into perspective, any work we do beyond a few hours a day is in excess to acquire more than we really need.

I've learned to consume less, spend less, and have less to avoid having to sell more and more of my time away to pay off things I've spent money on. Not only is this an eco green way to live, it also enables me to have more free time to spend with family, friends, work on projects that fill my soul, exercise, volunteer, make food to share, garden, and nap. For me, that's what defines wealth: owning my own time, health, happiness, and love.

HAPPY PLANET INDEX

Environmental implications, happiness, and well-being are measured per country by the Happy Planet Index (http://www.happyplanetindex.org/). It's been found that an increase in commute time decreases our level of happiness. Giving up your car, avoiding living alone, and shrugging off stress are some things that contribute to higher levels of happiness.

Flying has a terrible impact on the environment, and flying just six or seven hours uses up almost half our fair share of pollution for the entire year. To lighten your environmental footprint, instead of taking frequent, shorter holidays, consider fewer holidays where you visit for a longer time. And, consider taking the train instead of flying, if possible.

Desserts

Raw vegan desserts put me in a blissful state of happiness because I'm able to enjoy these without one ounce of guilt. All my recipes use superfoods like nuts, seeds, and fruits without refined sugar, butter, dairy, wheat, or gluten for a long and super life.

My desserts are good and good for you. They provide us with nutrients that build lean muscle mass and strong bones, boost the immune system, clear up the skin, and even help in losing extra unwanted pounds in a healthy way. My desserts will make you healthier from the inside out to give you a radiant glow of vitality and natural beauty that never fades.

The sweets of Southeast Asia are typically made from sticky rice and enjoyed between meals as snacks. Shaved ice is sweetened with syrup, fruit, and beans cooked in sugar. In India, sweets are dry or syrupy and use milk, almonds, pistachios, ghee, and sugar. Sweets are served at both the start and finish of a meal to help sweeten the palate.

China, Japan, and Korea traditionally enjoy sliced fresh fruits. Desserts in our home were always sliced apples or Asian pears. Simple, whole, fresh. The desserts in Korea are not as sweet as those in America; as a matter of fact, they are sometimes on the savory side. Today, bakeries popping up with cakes filled with red bean paste and mochi sweet rice cakes are popular.

Colonized countries in Asia have adopted custards like kheer in India. The Philippines has a leche flan, and Thailand has tapioca puddings. Even with the influence of the West, Asian desserts are not as heavy as Western desserts; many are fruit-based and use ingredients we consider more savory, like adzuki beans and corn.

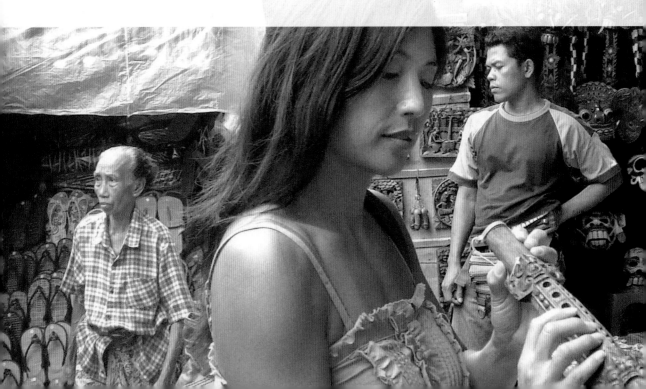

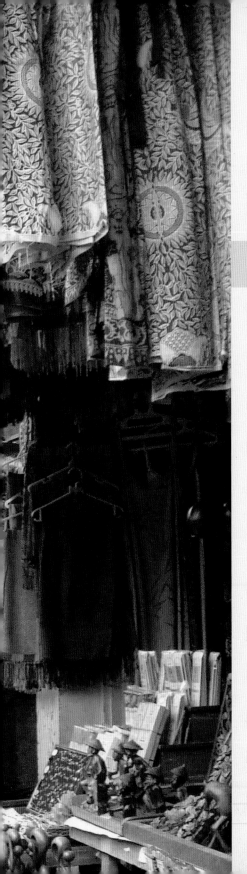

BUCKWHEAT CRISPIES

China

MAKES 2 CUPS

This recipe is from *Ani's Raw Food Kitchen*. Buckwheat is a seed that's free of wheat gluten. It's a great source of protein and is low in fat. To sprout buckwheat, see page 207.

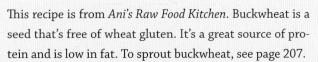

1 pound buckwheat groats

Soak groats in large mixing bowl in three times the amount of filtered water. Leave overnight. Rinse well the next morning. Drain.

Spread evenly on 14-inch square Excalibur Dehydrator mesh trays, and dry at 104°F for 3 to 5 hours, until completely dry.

Store in airtight glass jar. Will keep for several months.

HALO-HALO SHAVED ICE WITH COCONUT, FRUIT, CASHEW KREAM, AND MATCHA GREEN TEA ICE KREAM

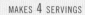
Philippines

MAKES 4 SERVINGS

This is a dessert popular in the Philippines. Fresh cubed fruits and legumes like adzuki beans are traditionally cooked in syrup until sweet and tender and are topped with shaved ice, ice cream, and milk. It's served with a long teaspoon and stirred continually as it's eaten. The flavors melt and mix together to create a new combination with each bite.

In my recipe, sweet corn, banana, coconut meat, mango, and jackfruit are topped with shaved ice, a sweet cashew mylk, scoop of ice kream, and Buckwheat Crispies. At first, the sweet corn may sound weird, but give it a try and expand your flavor palette. It's delicious as an interesting texture, color, and flavor.

Substitute any of the fruits in this recipe with cherries, crushed pineapple, papaya, or your favorite in-season fruit.

CASHEW MYLK

1 cup cashews

2 tablespoons agave or maple syrup

1 tablespoon alcohol-free vanilla extract

½ cup water, as desired

ICE

4 cups ice

TOPPING

1 batch Matcha Green Tea Ice Kream, page 261

½ cup Buckwheat Crispies, page 247

FRUITS

½ cup sweet corn kernels (about ½ ear of corn)

1 cup sliced banana (about 1 whole banana)

1 cup sliced Thai baby coconut meat

3 cups seeded, diced mango, cut into ½-inch cubes (about 2 to 3 whole mangos)

1 cup diced jackfruit, or substitute another fruit if unavailable

To make your mylk, add all ingredients into your blender. Blend smooth. Add as much water as needed for desired consistency. Set aside. I like a thicker kream consistency to mix with the melting shaved ice. I don't bother straining my mylks, I like the body the fiber gives.

Into four tall glasses or bowls, layer one-quarter of the corn, then banana, coconut, mango, and jackfruit into each.

To make your ice, place ice into food processor. Chop into tiny pieces.

To serve, use an ice cream scooper to tightly pack and scoop about ½ cup of shaved ice into each bowl. Pour ¼ cup mylk over each shaved ice and top with a scoop of ice cream. Sprinkle Buckwheat Crispies over it, and serve immediately.

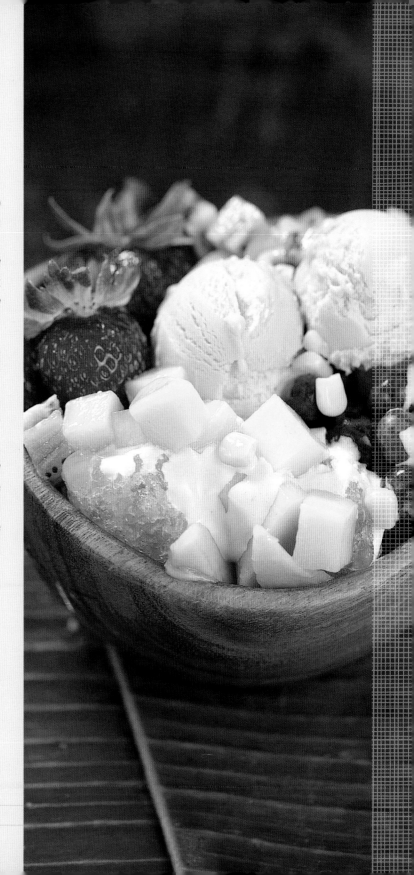

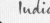

COCONUT BALLS IN SWEET ROSE KREAM WITH PISTACHIOS

India

MAKES 4 SERVINGS

This recipe is inspired by an Indian dessert called *Gulab Jamun*. It's a fried treat, sort of like a donut hole, that's soaked in a sweet syrup scented with rose water.

With this recipe, I blend almonds with rose water, cardamom, and coconut oil, then add coconut and oat flour to thicken. The dough is rolled into small balls and then served with a thinner version of my Cashew Mylk, made with rose water and topped with crushed pistachios.

This recipe calls for almond meal, which you can purchase, or better yet, just grind your own in a food processor. Don't over-process, or you'll end up with almond butter instead of powder.

MYLK

1 batch Cashew Mylk, page 44, made with rose water, or filtered water with a drop or 2 of rose extract

BATTER

½ cup almond meal

¼ cup agave syrup

1 tablespoon liquid coconut oil

½ teaspoon cardamom, powder

¼ teaspoon alcohol-free vanilla extract

2 to 3 tablespoons Rose Water, page 255, or filtered water with a drop or 2 of rose extract

FLOUR

½ cup oat flour, from about ½ cup ground oat groats

¾ cup coconut flour, from about 1 cup ground dry coconut

GARNISH

2 teaspoons chopped pistachios

2 teaspoons agave, brown rice, or maple syrup, or Date Syrup, page 43, optional

Make mylk by blending all ingredients smooth. Pour into a container, and set aside. No need to wash blender, just move to next step.

Place all batter ingredients into your high-speed blender. Blend smooth, adding only enough water as needed to blend a smooth, thick batter. Next, add flours to blender, and pulse to mix. Scrape out into a mixing bowl and mix by hand if needed, until mixed well. Form tablespoon-size balls and set aside.

To serve, pour about ⅓ cup of Cashew Mylk into each of four small dessert bowls. Next, place two coconut balls into each bowl. Sprinkle with pistachios and drizzle with agave syrup, if using. Enjoy immediately.

Balls will keep for several days stored on their own in the fridge.

VARIATION: *Make the coconut balls, then roll them in ¼ cup ground pistachios to make Gulab Jamun–inspired donut holes, without the mylk.*

CARDAMOM FOR GOOD HEALTH

Cardamom has a sweet, pleasant aroma that I love, and it's been used in Ayurveda to strengthen digestive activities as well as to balance the different constitutions defined as "doshas." Ayurveda is India's traditional, natural system of medicine practiced for more than five thousand years. *Ayurveda* is a Sanskrit word that means "practices of longevity."

In Chinese Medicine, cardamom is used to reduce air and water elements, increase appetite, and soothe mucous membranes. It relieves gas and heartburn, and a mix of cardamom, ginger, cloves, and coriander is a remedy for indigestion. Chewing cardamom seeds will also help dispel bad breath.

Cardamom has many other medicinal uses, including boiling in water with tea to remedy depression, as a daily gargle with cinnamon to protect against the flu, as an agent with cleansing and detoxifying properties, for soothing for asthma and bronchitis, and for nausea relief.

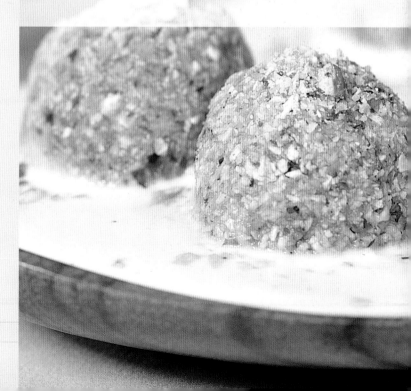

FIVE-SPICE POACHED PEARS PARFAIT WITH CANDIED WALNUTS

China

MAKES 4 SERVINGS

All five flavors of sour, bitter, sweet, pungent, and salty are found in Chinese Five Spice. Sweet ripe pears are sliced, drizzled with agave syrup, and seasoned with the sweet tones of star anise, cloves, and cinnamon with the bite of pepper, married with fennel seeds. The pear is placed in glasses between layers of Cashew Kream and Candied Walnuts.

You can use store-bought Five-Spice, or make your own with the following recipe on page 253.

If you don't have a dehydrator yet, you can use your oven set on the lowest heat. To keep this dish more raw, prop the door open with a spoon handle. It's hardly eco to dehydrate this way, but hopefully it will inspire you to invest in a dehydrator. They are fun to have and make crunchy, crispy textures that come only from drying.

CASHEW KREAM

2 batches Cashew Mylk, page 44, made using
    as little water as possible for a thicker
    kream texture

WALNUTS

1 cup walnuts

¼ cup agave or maple syrup

⅛ teaspoon sea salt

PEARS

2 ripe pears, soft to the touch, peeled,
    cored, sliced

1 teaspoon fresh lemon juice

2 tablespoons agave or maple syrup

½ teaspoon Chinese Five-Spice, page 253

Place walnuts, agave syrup, and salt into a bowl, and toss to mix and coat well. Spread onto a lined dehydrator tray, and dry at 104 degrees for 6 to 8 hours, or longer, to desired consistency.

Place sliced pears in a mixing bowl. Toss gently with lemon juice, then agave syrup. Coat well. Place slices onto a dehydrator tray and sprinkle with Chinese Five-Spice. Dry at 104°F for 6 to 8 hours, to desired consistency.

To serve, layer slices of pear into four parfait glasses, top with a scoop of Cashew Kream, sprinkle with walnuts, and then repeat layers. Enjoy immediately.

Will keep for a day in fridge.

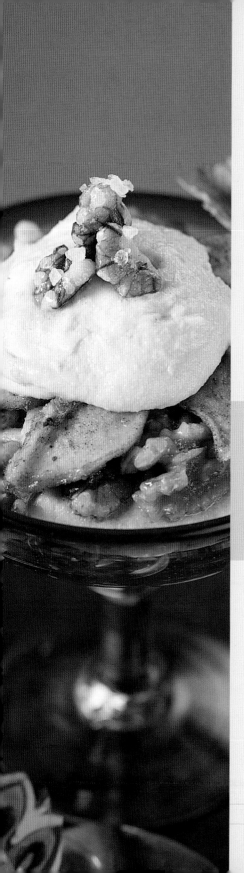

CHINESE FIVE-SPICE

China

MAKES ABOUT 3 TABLESPOONS

Typically, five-spice uses cinnamon (sweet), cloves (pungent, sweet), star anise (bitter), fennel (bitter like anise but sweeter and less pungent), and Szechuan peppercorns.

Szechuan peppercorns are not a pepper, but a berry. They taste peppery initially, then quickly numb the tongue, with hints of anise and ginger becoming lemony sour, salty, and hot. I use white ground pepper instead of Szechwan pepper in my recipe and add in ginger, bringing it technically to a Six-Spice.

Five-spice powder adds a spicy kick to rubs and marinades and is occasionally added to a sauce.

1½ tablespoons ground star anise

2½ teaspoons ground fennel seeds

1½ teaspoons ground cinnamon

½ teaspoon ground white pepper

½ teaspoon ground cloves

½ teaspoon ground ginger, optional

Mix together all spices.

Will keep for a month or more stored in an airtight container at room temperature.

SAFFRON CARDAMOM CASHEW "RICE" PUDDING WITH ROSE WATER

India

MAKES 4 SERVINGS

I love saffron, a popular but expensive Indian spice that is the actual stigma, or female part, of a species of crocus. More than 150,000 flowers and 400 hours of labor only yield 2 pounds of saffron. The flavor is strong, tastes bittersweet, and is somewhat sharp so you only need to use a tiny bit in recipes. It's available dried, ground, or crushed; I look for the whole dried strands.

I use a mix of small rice-size pieces of cashew folded into a Cashew Kream to make my rice pudding. The kream is seasoned with a few strands of saffron—which adds a rich yellow color—cardamom and rose water. This pudding is great as a dessert, snack, and for breakfast.

You can find distilled rose water in a bottle at an Indian or Middle Eastern grocery. Or, you can make your own with the recipe that follows on page 255.

To serve your pudding warm, place it in a bowl and put the bowl in your dehydrator for a few hours at 104°F. If you don't have a dehydrator yet, you can use your oven set on the lowest heat.

KREAM

2 cups cashews

2 tablespoons agave or maple syrup

¼ teaspoon saffron threads

¼ teaspoon cardamom powder

1 cup Rose Water, see page 255

RICE

2 cups pistachios

⅛ teaspoon sea salt

TOPPING

¼ cup slivered almonds

2 tablespoons chopped pistachios

2 teaspoons ground cinnamon

To make your rice, place pistachio and salt into a food processor and process into small, rice-size pieces. Avoid over-processing into powder. Set aside.

To make kream, place all ingredients into your blender, adding just enough water to make a thick kream texture. Scoop into a bowl, and stir in the pistachio rice pieces.

To serve, scoop into four bowls. Top with slivered almonds, pistachios, and cinnamon.

Will keep for 3 to 4 days in fridge.

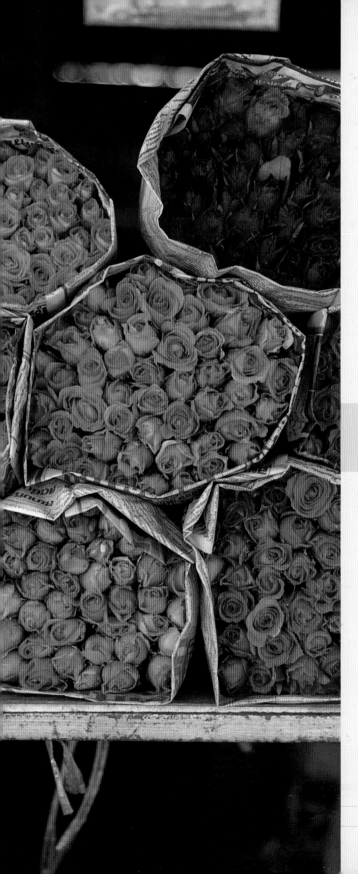

ROSE WATER

India

MAKES ABOUT 1 CUP

To make this recipe, use freshly picked rose petals free of chemical pesticides or chemicals and, ideally, organic. Use only the petals and not the stems or leaves. Wash the petals by submerging in a bowl of water to remove bugs or dirt and use immediately.

Rose water works great as a facial toner or astringent, as well as adding a fragrant flavor to food.

½ cup firmly packed rose petals
1 cup filtered water

Blend petals and water for at least a minute. Pour through a sieve to strain out the petals and squeeze out the remaining liquid from the petals.

Store immediately in a sealed jar in the fridge. Best to use as soon as possible, if not immediately. Batches vary and may last a few days or longer.

VANILLA CINNAMON "RICE" PUDDING WITH COCONUT MILK AND SLICED BANANA

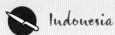

Indonesia

MAKES 4 SERVINGS

A pudding eaten by the Balinese as an afternoon snack called *Bubur Injin*. The cooked recipe uses a black rice and calls for pandan leaf as a spice to add a somewhat nutty and pleasant plant aroma. Pandan isn't very easy to find, so I use vanilla in my recipe instead of the pandan.

RICE

1 batch Cashew Nut "Rice," page 221

2 tablespoons agave syrup

2 tablespoons alcohol-free vanilla extract or 2 vanilla beans, seeded

½ teaspoon cinnamon

GARNISH

2 batches Coconut Milk, page 144

1 tablespoon agave or maple syrup, optional

1 cup sliced banana

1 tablespoon shredded coconut

Make rice by placing all ingredients into food processor. Pulse lightly to mix.

To serve, scoop rice into four serving bowls. If using agave syrup, mix with coconut milk. Pour about ½ cup of milk around the rice in each bowl. Top with sliced banana and shredded coconut. Enjoy immediately.

Will keep for 2 days in fridge.

ASIAN BLACK "RICE" CHIA PUDDING

Indonesia

MAKES 4 SERVINGS

Popular for breakfast in parts of Southeast Asia and a delicious dessert. Traditionally Thai black sticky rice or a Chinese black rice, sometimes called forbidden rice, is cooked and then sugar, pinch of salt, and coconut milk are stirred in and brought to a boil. The texture is thick and slightly chewy.

Chia seeds are small black seeds that when mixed with water, become a gel. Mixed with your favorite nut mylk, chia seeds create a texture similar to tapioca pudding. Chia seeds are hydrophilic, they absorb more than twelve times their weight in water, hold on to water, and help hydrate us. The seeds are said to be the highest source of essential omega-3 fatty acid and are a rich source of calcium.

1 batch Nut and Seed Mylk, page 44
½ cup chia seeds

Place chia seeds into a bowl and add about 4 cups of mylk. Set aside for 10 minutes or longer, and the chia will soak up the liquid and create a thick gel. Add more mylk if preferred.

To serve, scoop into four serving bowls. Top with a splash of mylk.

Pudding will keep for a day or two in fridge.

VARIATIONS: *Try adding a tablespoon of cacao, carob powder, or vanilla extract. Add spices like cinnamon or cardamom and add sliced fresh fruit like banana, pear, kiwi, or berries. Or, add dry fruits and nuts like goji berries, walnuts, and pecans and top with Coconut Milk, page 144. Serve with Chocolate Syrup, page 267.*

SWEET SESAME HALVAH

Korea

MAKES ABOUT 16 CANDIES

A candy reminiscent of American peanut butter balls and Middle Eastern Halvah. You can use a plastic chocolate candy mold or a shell-shaped French mini Madeline cake tin, or just roll the dough into little balls. Makes pretty gifts when packed into candy cups and a decorative box or recycled jar tied with a ribbon.

Almond butters will have stiffer or runnier textures, so if your batter is less firm than you like, add more sesame seeds to help stiffen it up. If you don't have yacon syrup, start with half the amount of agave syrup and adjust to your liking.

½ cup sesame seeds, lightly crushed in a mortar and pestle or grinder

½ cup almond butter

¼ cup yacon syrup

½ teaspoon sea salt

Into a food processor, place all ingredients. Pulse to mix into a texture similar to a chunky peanut butter.

Place a sheet of plastic wrap over your mold, if using. Take a tablespoon or two, depending on the size of your candy mold, and press into the plastic wrap and into the mold firmly. You can also roll into tablespoon-size balls without a mold. Place into freezer 10 minutes to chill.

Remove from freezer and gently lift plastic wrap up to release candies from molds.

Store in airtight container in freezer. Will keep for a couple of weeks.

VARIATION: *Use tahini instead of almond butter. Tahini comes in various consistencies too, so adjust by adding more sesame seeds if you need to stiffen it up.*

LYCHEE ASIAN LIME CREPES WITH GINGER PEAR SORBET

Thailand

MAKES 4 SERVINGS

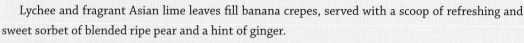

Lychees are round and about 1½ inches in diameter. They're covered by a reddish, roughly textured, and thin skin that's easy to peel away. The fruit inside is translucent, sweet, juicy, and rich in vitamin C.

Lychee and fragrant Asian lime leaves fill banana crepes, served with a scoop of refreshing and sweet sorbet of blended ripe pear and a hint of ginger.

Lychee are available during the summer at Asian grocery stores. If you can't find lychees, use your favorite fruit instead like pears, bananas, kiwi, and or berries.

 If you don't have a dehydrator yet, you can use your oven set on the lowest heat to dry your crepes on a baking tray. To keep this dish more raw, prop the door open with a spoon handle.

CREPES (FROM *ANI'S RAW FOOD ESSENTIALS*, PAGE 68)

2 cups sliced and packed tightly banana (about 4 whole bananas)

1 cup flax meal

1 cup filtered water, as needed

FILLING

3 cups peeled, seeded, diced, and drained lychee

½ teaspoon julienned Asian lime leaf

GINGER PEAR SORBET

2 cups peeled, chopped, frozen Anjou or Bartlett pears (about 2 large)

½ cup filtered water, as needed

⅓ cup agave syrup

1 teaspoon grated ginger

To make your crepes, place banana into bottom of your blender. Top with flax meal and water, blend smooth. Spread batter evenly onto two lined 14-inch dehydrator trays. Dry at 104°F for 4 to 6 hours, until completely dry. Cut each sheet into two pieces for a total of four crepes.

To make sorbet, combine all ingredients in high-speed blender. Use as little water as possible to blend smooth. The less water you use, the less icy your sorbet will be. Scoop mixture into ice cream maker to firm up, or just scoop into a container and place into freezer for an hour or more to firm up.

To serve, place a crepe rectangle onto a flat surface. Fill with lychee, sprinkle on lime leaf, and roll up. Top with a scoop of Ginger Pear Sorbet. Enjoy immediately.

MOCHI COCONUT MAKI ROLLS
WITH CHOCOLATE FUDGE SAUCE

Japan

MAKES 6 TO 8 SERVINGS

Coconut Wrappers have a similar texture to mochi when
used in this sweet recipe. Roll up your favorite ice kream
inside wrappers to make a beautiful mochi- and maki-in-
spired dessert. Serve with a side of Chocolate Fudge Sauce
for dipping.

1 batch Chocolate Fudge Sauce, page 52

1 batch Coconut Wrappers, page 178, cut into a total of
4 rectangles (2 per tray)

1 batch Matcha Green Tea Ice Kream (page 261), Coconut
Vanilla Goji Berry (page 264), Chai (page 266), or your
favorite Ice Kream

To serve, scoop Chocolate Fudge Sauce into four small sauce bowls.
Set aside.

Lay Coconut Wrapper on flat surface. Spread ½ cup of ice kream
evenly across wrapper. Roll up from bottom and then slice into
rounds. Serve immediately with Chocolate Fudge Sauce or place in
container and store in freezer until ready to eat.

Will keep for many days in freezer, but best enjoyed immediately.

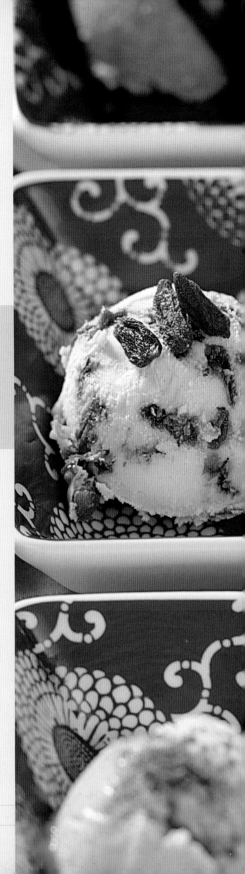

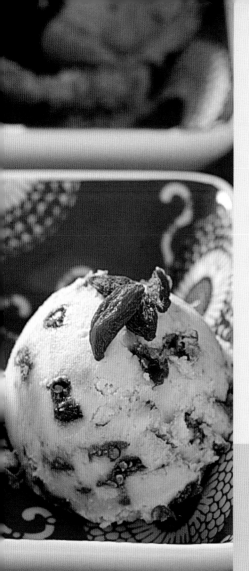

MATCHA GREEN TEA ICE KREAM

Japan

MAKES 1 ½ CUPS

Matcha is a bright green powder made from destemmed, deveined, stone-ground, and shade-grown green tea leaves. It's exponentially higher in antioxidants than blueberries and spinach. Matcha is a chlorophyll (green pigment)–rich food since the whole leaf is ingested when consumed, and it helps remove heavy metals and chemical toxins from the body. It's naturally mood enhancing, sugar-free, and high in fiber.

This beautiful green ice kream is made by blending sweet cashews with vanilla, agave syrup, and matcha green tea powder. The agave syrup doesn't freeze solid in the cold, and it will keep this ice kream scoopable out of the freezer.

1 cup cashews

4 to 6 teaspoons green tea powder, to taste

1 tablespoon alcohol-free vanilla extract

¼ cup agave syrup

4 to 6 tablespoons Coconut Milk, page 144, as needed, or filtered water

To make your ice kream, place all ingredients into your high-speed blender, adding only enough water as needed to blend into a smooth cream texture.

Scoop into ice cream maker, if using. Or just scoop into a container and place in freezer overnight to firm up.

Will keep for at least a week in your freezer.

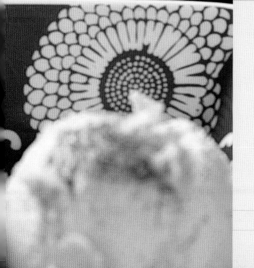

LAVENDER ICE KREAM WITH BLACKBERRY JAM, LAVENDER SYRUP, AND CASHEW KREAM ON BUCKWHEAT BISCUIT

Indonesia

MAKES 4 SERVINGS

My friends and I ordered this beautiful dessert in Nusa Dua, Bali, at a 5-star resort. It was made with dairy cream and lots of sugar. When I saw it, I realized how easy it would be to make a healthy, vegan, raw version of the same dessert.

If you don't have a dehydrator yet, you can use your oven set on the lowest heat. To keep this dish more raw, prop the door open with a spoon handle. It's hardly eco to dehydrate this way, but hopefully it will inspire you to invest in a dehydrator. Or, just skip the biscuit and enjoy the rest of the flavors together in a bowl.

BISCUIT

1 cup buckwheat, soaked 8 to 12 hours, rinse well

2 tablespoons liquid coconut oil

2 tablespoons agave syrup

⅔ cup filtered water, as needed

2 tablespoons ground into meal (powder) golden flaxseed

LAVENDER SYRUP (FROM *ANI'S RAW FOOD DESSERTS*, PAGE 172)

2 tablespoons fresh lavender flowers or 1 tablespoon dried

½ cup agave syrup

LAVENDER ICE KREAM

1 cup cashews

1 tablespoon alcohol-free vanilla extract

¼ cup Lavender Syrup

4 to 6 tablespoons Coconut Milk, page 144, as needed, or filtered water

BLACKBERRY JAM

1 cup blackberries

¼ cup pitted, packed Medjool dates

CASHEW KREAM

1 batch Cashew Mylk, page 44, made using as little water as possible for a thicker kream texture

To make biscuits, in your high speed blender place soaked and rinsed buckwheat, coconut oil, agave syrup, and just enough water to blend into smooth, thick cream texture. Add flax meal with just enough water to mix smooth. Scoop batter into ¼-cup biscuit shapes on a lined dehydrator tray. Dry for 8 to 10 hours at 104°F.

To make syrup, blend lavender flowers and agave syrup in small blender for 30 seconds or longer, making sure syrup doesn't get too hot. Set aside.

To make ice kream, place all ingredients into your high-speed blender, adding only enough water as needed to blend into a smooth cream texture. Scoop into ice cream maker, if using. Or just scoop into a container and place in freezer overnight to firm up.

To make jam, place blueberries and dates into food processor. Pulse lightly into chunky jam consistency. Set aside.

To serve, scoop 1 tablespoon Lavender Syrup in center at bottom of each of four dessert bowls or plates. Place biscuit on top of syrup. Top biscuit with Cashew Kream, blueberry jam, and a scoop of Lavender Ice Kream. Serve immediately.

THROUGH THE EYES OF A CHILD

The other night was a friend's birthday celebration. He wanted to see a Pink Floyd cover band at a big venue in the Valley outside Los Angeles, which was something I'd never choose to do myself. Rather than focus on all the bad points (like how it would take two hours in Friday rush-hour traffic to get there, how I don't watch much music other than DJs on turntables, and how uncool it was to party in the Valley when I live right in the heart of West Hollywood) I decided to keep an open mind, just like a child would. A child can do the same thing day after day, like swing on the same swing set. But each time, it's as if it's her very first time.

Approaching life as a child, seeing things for the first time, means leaving room for surprises. Rather than being a know-it-all, keeping a sense of wonder and awe means I usually discover something new and exciting. In the case of the Pink Floyd cover band, I met several amazing people who are now my dear friends. I danced up a storm and had a blast. I also discovered this was a venue where 80s bands still play, like The English Beat, whom I love and who were playing just a few weeks later.

COCONUT VANILLA GOJI BERRY ICE KREAM

China

MAKES ABOUT 2 CUPS

Coconut meat and cashews are blended to create a smooth, rich, ice kream texture. Then, red gojis are folded through for a beautiful, delicious, vitamin C and protein packed frozen treat. The agave syrup won't freeze up and is what keeps this ice kream scoopable straight out of the freezer, no thawing required.

1 cup goji berries

1 cup coconut meat

¾ cup cashews

¼ cup agave syrup

1 vanilla bean, scraped, or 1 tablespoon alcohol-free vanilla extract

¼ cup liquid coconut oil

First, place goji berries into a bowl with about a cup of filtered water, making sure all berries are submerged. Set aside for 20 to 30 minutes to hydrate and soften. Squeeze out excess water by hand before using.

Into your high-speed blender, place coconut meat first, then cashews, agave syrup, vanilla, and coconut oil. Blend smooth. Add soaked and drained goji berries and pulse once only to mix. Do not over-mix, or your ice kream will turn pink.

Scoop into ice cream maker, if using, and follow manufacturer's instructions. Or, just scoop into a container and place in freezer overnight to firm up.

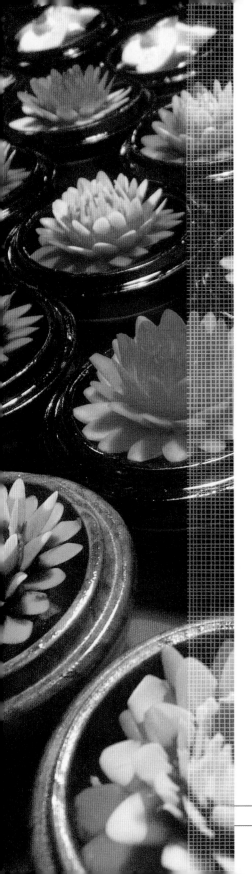

GOJI BERRIES FOR LONGEVITY

Goji berries have been used in Chinese Medicine for a few thousand years. Today, more than fifty clinical studies list over thirty reasons to consume goji berries including enhancing sexuality; weight loss; relief from headaches, dizziness, and insomnia; lowering the risk of cancer; and promoting normal blood sugar.

In Chinese Medicine, goji berries are believed to enhance immune system function, improve eyesight, protect the liver, improve circulation, and enrich yin. In China, it's advised for people who work at computers to drink herbal tea made from goji berries and chrysanthemum, since gojis are good for our eyes.

Goji berries contain nineteen amino acids, twenty-one trace minerals, more protein than whole wheat, and higher levels of vitamin C than oranges. Goji berries have been used to rejuvenate cells, protect against germs, relieve arthritis, and help alleviate depression and sexual dysfunction.

Tibetan and Chinese legends tell of people who've lived century-long lives while retaining the strength and beauty of youth, thanks to the goji berry.

CHAI ICE KREAM WITH CHOCOLATE SYRUP

India

MAKES 2 CUPS

Chai is an Indian milk tea that's recently made its way to coffee- and teahouses throughout the United States. The flavor of this ice kream comes from ginger, cardamom, cinnamon, and vanilla, sweetened with a whole fruit, dates. I recommend using a semi-soft variety like Medjool or honey date. You can use a drier date, but you will need to add more coconut water to compensate.

When blending, try to use the least amount of water as possible. The less water you add, the less ice crystals you'll have in your frozen ice kream.

1 cup ripe banana, about 2 whole

1 cup cashews

2 vanilla beans, scraped, or 2 tablespoons alcohol-free vanilla extract

¼ teaspoon ground cardamom

¼ teaspoon ground cinnamon

Pinch of ground clove, to taste

1 cup Thai baby coconut water, or Coconut Milk, page 144, or filtered water, as needed

½ cup pitted, packed Medjool dates

SYRUP

1 batch Chocolate Syrup, page 267

Into blender, place banana, cashews, vanilla, cardamom, cinnamon, clove, and only enough coconut water needed to blend into a smooth cream. Add dates and blend to mix well, adding more water if needed.

Scoop into an ice cream maker, if using, and follow the manufacturer's instructions. Or just scoop into a container and place in freezer overnight to firm up. You may need to thaw for 5 or 10 minutes before scooping.

Serve with Chocolate Syrup.

KREAMY SHAVED ICE WITH FRESH FRUIT AND CHOCOLATE SYRUP

Korea

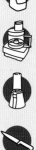

MAKES 4 SERVINGS

Patbingsu is a Korean shaved ice dessert loaded with sweet toppings like chopped fruit, condensed milk, fruit syrup, and red adzyki beans. *Pat* means "red beans" and *bingsu* is shaved ice.

This recipe layers fruit on top of chopped ice with Cashew Mylk and Chocolate Syrup.

Patbingsu is most fun when eaten in pairs where two friends, family members, or lovers typically share a bowl together. It's possible to find an ice-shaving machine at a Korean market for about $40, but I just chop up my ice cubes in a food processor instead.

Feel free to substitute your favorite in-season fruits like lychee, rambutan, tangerine, berries, pomegranate, or pineapple.

MYLK
1 batch Cashew Mylk, page 44

CHOCOLATE SYRUP
½ cup cacao powder
½ cup agave, maple, or Date Syrup, page 43
1 teaspoon extra-virgin olive oil or coconut oil

FRUITS
2 cups sliced peaches and/or pears and/or apricots
1 cup sliced kiwi
1 cup sliced banana
1 cup ½-inch-cubed melon

ICE
4 cups ice

To make your Chocolate Syrup, place all ingredients into a small blender. Blend smooth. If using a larger blender, double the recipe to ensure the blender blades are covered. If using Date Syrup, you may want to add a splash of filtered water to thin out the consistency, or not. Set aside.

Before serving, make sure all your fruit is ready to go. Then, "shave" your ice by placing ice into food processor. Chop into tiny pieces. Use an ice cream scooper to tightly pack and scoop about 1 cup of shaved ice into each of two bowls, if sharing in pairs, which I recommend.

Into each of your two bowls, pour ½ cup mylk over the ice. Then, top with half of the fruit. Drizzle on your Chocolate Syrup. Serve with two spoons in each bowl to be enjoyed immediately.

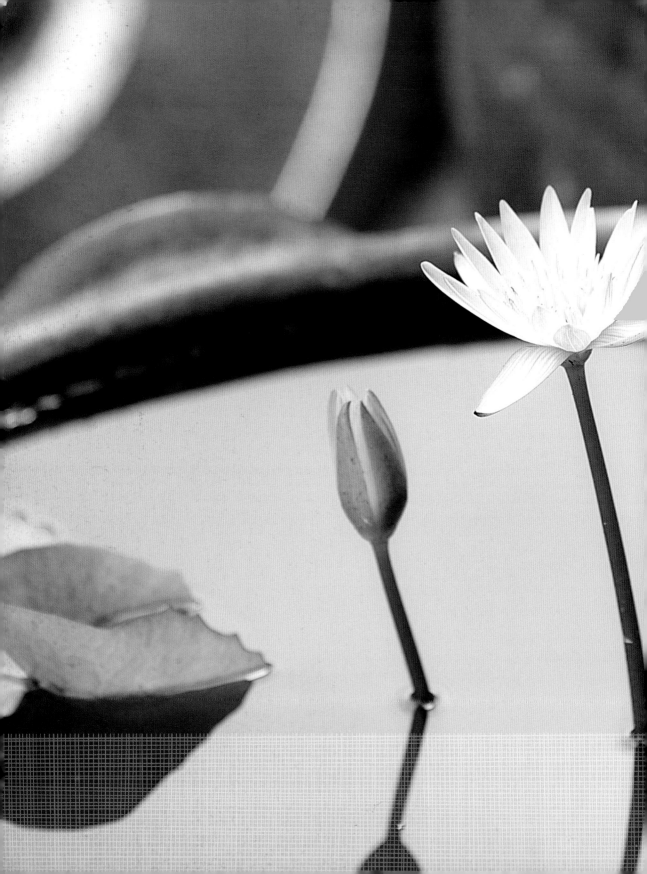

10

menus

Use these sample menus to help plan a brunch, a cocktail party, a dinner, a picnic, a birthday party, and all types of celebrations, even a wedding. I'll point out a bunch of Asian aphrodisiacs and love-life ingredients like ginger, durian fruit, vanilla, and wine, because we can always add more love into our lives, right? And I also include recipes that work well buffet-style, for potlucks, and as take-home gifts.

Menus for Entertaining

BRUNCH

Weekend brunches are a great way to kick off a relaxing day with friends and family. Most of the menu items for brunch can be prepared the day before so you can still sleep in before your guests arrive. The dehydrated recipes can be tossed into your dehydrator the night before and served warm.

BRUNCH, KOREA
Nut and Seed Mylk, page 44

Cinnamon, Fig, and Ginger Sun Tea, page 47

Scallion Pancakes with Spicy Sesame Oil Dipping Sauce, page 182

Kreamy Shaved Ice with Fresh Fruit and Chocolate Syrup, page 267

BRUNCH, INDONESIA
Avocado Shake with Optional Chocolate Fudge Sauce, page 51

Corn Fritters with a Hot and Sour Cucumber Dipping Sauce, page 176

Vanilla Cinnamon "Rice" Pudding with Coconut Milk and Sliced Banana, page 256

BRUNCH, INDIA
Mango Lassi, page 52

Samosas with Tomato Dal, page 168

Saffron Cardamom Cashew "Rice" Pudding with Rose Water, page 254

BRUNCH, CHINA
Nut and Seed Mylks, page 44

Five-Spice Poached Pears Parfait with Candied Walnuts, page 252

Moo Shoo Vegetables with Hoisin Sauce, page 180

COCKTAIL PARTIES

*Raw*ktail parties are a great way to celebrate life, love, friends, and good fortune. Serve any or all of the beautiful cocktails and/or shakes in the Drinks chapter alongside these easy-to-snack-on finger foods.

Cilantro Cheeze–Stuffed Cucumber Ravioli, page 123

Lotus Root Chips with Pine Nut Mustard Sauce, page 124

Mixed Vegetable Skewers with Almond Butter Sauce, page 117

Vegetable Tempura with Orange Lemongrass Dipping Sauce, page 118

Iceberg Lettuce Wraps with Mock Tamarind Sauce, page 165

Summer Rolls with Ginger "Peanut" Sauce, page 170

Mixed Vegetable Seaweed Rolls, page 233

Mixed Vegetable Nori Rolls with Pickled Ginger and Wasabi, page 234

Samosas with Tomato Dal, page 168

Corn Fritters with a Hot and Sour Cucumber Dipping Sauce, page 176

Spring Rolls with Mango Dipping Sauce, page 184

Sweet Sesame Halvah, page 258

Coconut Balls with Pistachios, rolled in pistachio, serve as donut holes without the mylk, page 251

DINNER PARTIES

I love an air of sophistication, elegance, and complexity for my dinner parties. The full flavors of my recipes may make it seem as though I've spent days in my kitchen preparing, but these recipes are quick and easy to put together. Serve dinner with your favorite biodynamic wines.

DINNER, KOREA

Pomegranate Cocktail, page 55

Sesame Romaine Salad, page 62

Cucumber Kimchi, page 92

Bi-Bim-Bop (Mixed Vegetable "Rice"), page 224

Sweet Sesame Halvah, page 258

Sliced fresh fruit, like apple, Asian pear, persimmons

DINNER, JAPAN

Blushing Roses, page 56

Black and Tan Encrusted Coconut Meat on a Bed of Shredded Daikon, Carrots, and Cucumbers Tossed in Goddess Dressing, page 78

Noodles in Clear Seaweed Broth with Japanese Seven-Spice, page 210

Matcha Green Tea Ice Kream, page 261

DINNER, THAILAND

Coconut Tomato Soup, page 143

Green Mango and Coconut Noodle Salad, page 66

Pineapple "Fried Rice" with Pineapple Curry Sauce, page 226

Lychee Asian Lime Crepes with Ginger Pear Sorbet, page 259

PICNICS

Eating and sharing food outside on a blanket in the park on a sunny summer late afternoon or evening is one of my favorite pastimes. The following recipes travel well and can stay out of the fridge for several hours.

SOUPS

Coconut Hot and Sour Soup with Mixed Marinated Mushrooms, page 145

Seaweed Soup with Shiitake and Daikon, page 139

SALADS

Green Papaya Salad, page 70

Pineapple, Red Cabbage, and Corn Salad, page 74

Carrot, Cucumber, and Red Bell Pepper Matchstick Salad, page 67

All pickles and namuls, pages 82–104

VEGETABLES

Kreamed Curry Saag Spinach, page 111

Mixed Vegetable Skewers with Almond Butter Sauce, page 117

Yellow Coconut Curry Vegetables, page 150

Lotus Root Chips with Pine Nut Mustard Sauce, page 124

Vegetable Tempura with Orange Lemongrass Dipping Sauce, page 118

Samosas with Tomato Dal, page 168

Scallion Pancakes with Spicy Sesame Oil Dipping Sauce, page 182

NOODLES

Spicy Mixed Vegetable Noodles, page 200

Noodles and Vegetables in a Red Curry Sauce, page 208

RICE

Jicama "Rice" with Sliced Scallions and Sesame Oil, page 222

Coconut Saffron "Rice" with Tomato Mango Sambal, page 228

Sweet Corn "Rice" with Lemongrass Chili, page 220

DESSERT

Coconut Balls with Pistachios, rolled in pistachio, serve as donut holes without the mylk,
    page 251

Asian Black "Rice" Chia Pudding, page 257

Sweet Sesame Halvah, page 258

BIRTHDAYS AND CELEBRATIONS

The best desserts for celebrating are raw desserts—after all, they're made with superfoods that fuel a Super Life. As you already know, they are guilt-free and good for our health. Serve any and all of the desserts in this book at your next birthday party or celebration.

WEDDINGS

Someone once asked me to help add in my raw dishes to a fully catered wedding menu to offer a few healthier options. Below are sample menus, but any of the following recipes can be added onto an existing menu.

WEDDING A

Coconut Durian Shake, page 49

Spring Rolls with Mango Dipping Sauce, page 184

Pineapple, Red Cabbage, and Corn Salad, page 74

Green Papaya Soup, page 146

Coconut Saffron "Rice" with Tomato Mango Sambal, page 228
Coconut Balls in Sweet Rose Kream with Pistachios, page 250

WEDDING B

Mango Lassi, page 52
Green Papaya Salad, page 70
Cilantro Cheeze–Stuffed Cucumber Ravioli, page 123
Pineapple "Fried Rice" with Pineapple Curry Sauce, page 226
Chai Ice Kream with Chocolate Syrup, page 266

WEDDING C

Green Mango and Coconut Noodle Salad, page 66
Summer Rolls with Ginger "Peanut" Sauce, page 170
Baby Bok Choy with Chinese Cabbage in Ginger Sauce, page 113
Noodles and Vegetables in a Red Curry Sauce, page 208
Vanilla Cinnamon "Rice" Pudding with Coconut Milk and Sliced Banana, page 256

BUFFETS AND POTLUCKS

For buffets and potlucks, dishes that can be quickly prepared in volume, several batches at a time, and served family-style in a large serving bowl or platter work best. Any or all of these dishes will keep fine sitting out for several hours.

SALAD

Green Mango and Coconut Noodle Salad, page 64
Green Papaya Salad, page 70

VEGETABLES

All pickles and namuls, pages 82–104
Mixed Vegetable Skewers with Almond Butter Sauce, page 117
Kreamed Curry Saag Spinach, page 111

SOUP

Miso Soup with Spinach and Bean Sprouts, page 136
Sesame Mushroom Soup, page 138
Coconut Tomato Soup, page 143

NOODLES

Spicy Mixed Vegetable Noodles, page 200

Glass Noodles with Marinated Mushrooms, Spinach, and Carrots, page 201

RICE

Jicama "Rice" with Sliced Scallions and Sesame Oil, page 222

Coconut Saffron "Rice" with Tomato Mango Sambal, page 228

Sweet Corn "Rice" with Lemongrass Chili, page 220

Vanilla Cinnamon "Rice" Pudding with Coconut Milk and Sliced Banana, page 256

DESSERT

Five-Spice Poached Pears Parfait with Candied Walnuts, page 252

Saffron Cardamom Cashew "Rice" Pudding with Rose Water, page 254

ROMANTIC DINNERS

Serve any of the Wedding menus, page 273, for your special dinner for two. Add in some cocktails from the Drinks chapter or your favorite bottle of biodynamic wine.

TAKE-HOME GIFTS

At the close of a celebration, I like to give guests a treat they can take home to carry the feeling of love, happiness, and gratitude into the days that follow. These items keep fine for a few hours until your guest can get them into their fridge at home.

Pickles, in a jar with ribbon, stickers, and/or label, pages 82–85

Kimchi, in a jar with ribbon, stickers, and/or label, pages 87–92

Saffron Cardamom Cashew "Rice" Pudding with Rose Water, in single-serving container with ribbon, page 254

Coconut Balls with Pistachios, rolled in pistachio, serve as donut holes without the mylk, packaged in a small container or bag, tied with ribbon, page 251

Sweet Sesame Halvah, packaged in small container or a bag, tied with ribbon, page 258

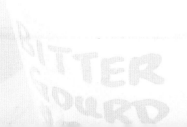

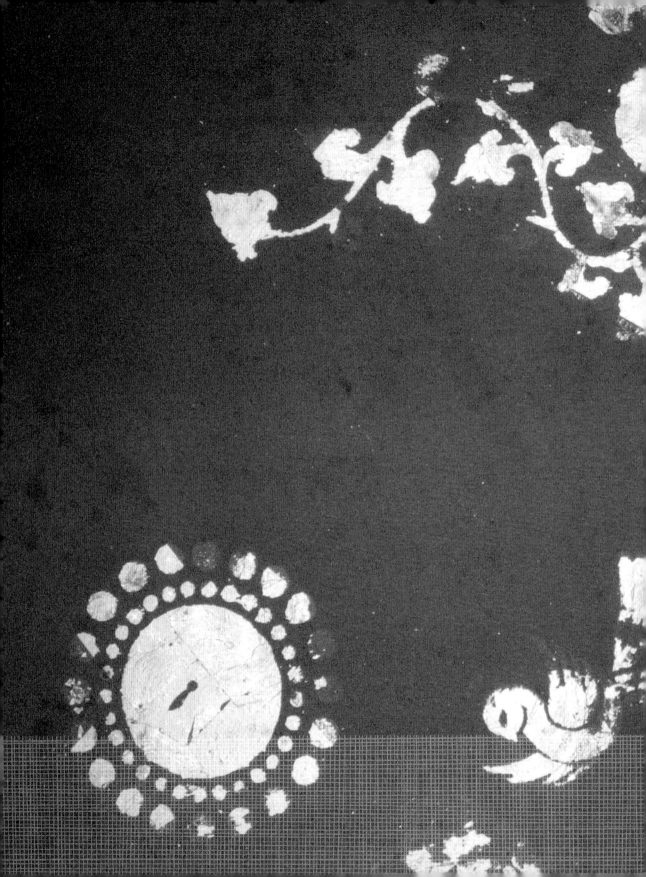

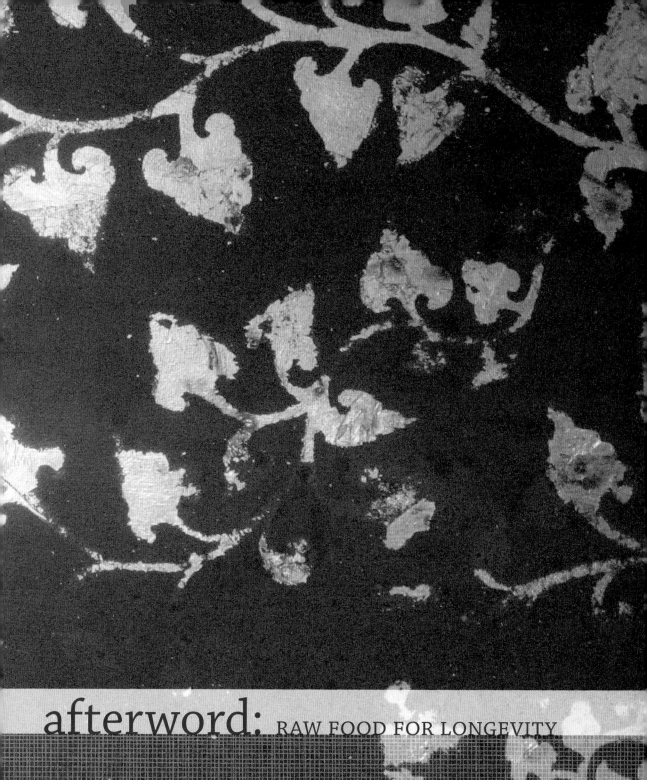

afterword: RAW FOOD FOR LONGEVITY

Theories on Longevity

I've come across several interesting theories on longevity. They include oxygenated environments, lowering our caloric intake, grazing throughout the day, eating nutrient-rich foods, lifestyle, and genetics. The Okinawans are known to have the longest lifespan—they age slowly while delaying and avoiding chronic diseases of aging like dementia, heart disease, stroke, and cancer.

OKINAWA CENTENARIAN STUDY

This study was started in 1976 by Makoto Suzuki, M.D., Ph.D. (cardiologist and geriatrician); Bradley Willcox M.D., M.S. (physician-investigator in geriatrics), and Craig Willcox, Ph.D. (healthy aging expert). They documented over nine hundred Okinawan centenarians along with other elderly people in their seventies, eighties, and nineties to find that genetic factors play a role in helping prevent inflammatory and autoimmune diseases, and about a third of our human lifespan may be heritable. These centenarians and near-centenarians lived within the same families and many were siblings. But, when Okinawans moved to a new environment and changed their lifestyle habits, they lost their longevity. So, not all Okinawan longevity can be contributed to genetics. Their lifestyle plays an even larger role in their longevity.

One theory says that aging is caused by stress we put on our bodies in digesting food we eat to create energy. Digestion creates free radicals, which are unstable molecules that damage body tissue, DNA, and other vital body molecules. This damage adds up over time and degenerates our body. This wear and tear on our system can be lessened by eating fewer calories. The Okinawans eat a low-calorie diet and eat only to 80 percent fullness. In turn, they have low levels of free radicals in their blood and healthier hearts, and they are at lower risk for cancer and chronic diseases.

The Okinawan seniors were found to have young, clean arteries and low cholesterol levels, especially compared to Westerners, due to their diet, regular exercise, positive outlook, low-stress lifestyle, moderate alcohol use, and avoidance of smoking. An autopsy of a centenarian showed completely plaque-free arteries. The study also discovered that higher levels of folate in the diet (from dark leafy vegetables) meant lower levels of heart disease.

A low-calorie and low-glycemic diet consisting of high levels of vegetables, fruits, and good fats like omega-3, high fiber, plus low body fat and high levels of physical activity throughout their long lives protect Okinawans from heart disease, stroke, and cancers. They have 80 percent less breast cancer and prostate cancer and 50 percent less ovarian and colon cancers than Westerners. Okinawan centenarians are lean throughout their lives, with an average body mass index between 18 to 22. They also demonstrated healthy cognitive aging, with low levels of dementia due to their positive outlook, low-stress lifestyle, strong ability to cope, sense of meaning and purpose, and spiritual practice.

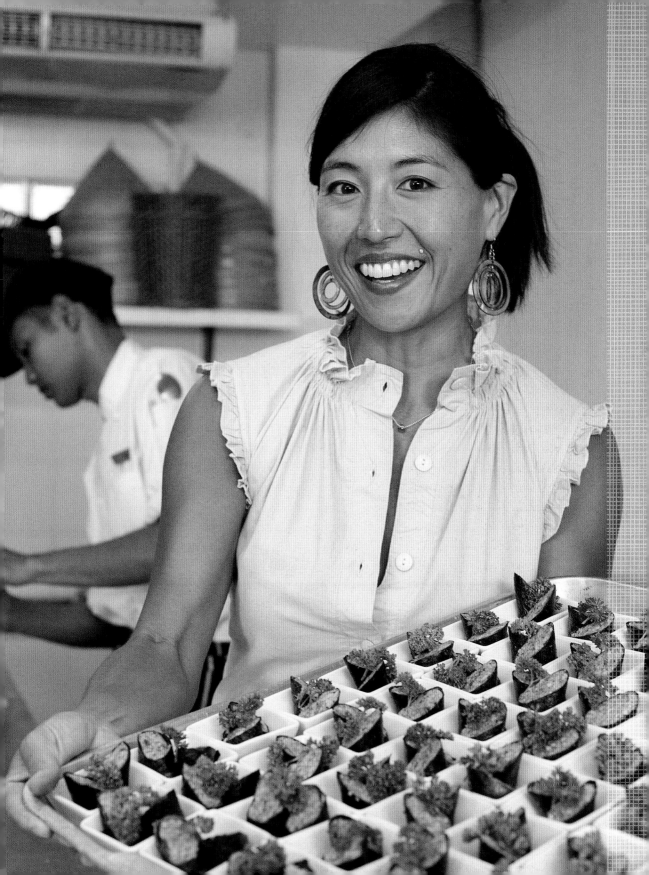

Bone density in the elderly Okinawans remained at healthy levels for long periods of time. They had 40 percent less hip factures than Americans, and their high calcium intake from water and food, high vitamin D from sunlight, high levels of physical activity through older ages, and high levels of flavonoids in their diet from plant foods protected their bones.

Estrogen, testosterone, and DHEA were found in higher levels in Okinawan elders than Americans, suggesting they age much slower than Americans, and in comparison, are physically younger. (Dehydroepiandrosterone [DHEA], a hormone made in the human body and secreted by the adrenal gland, is a precursor to sex hormones in men and women. DHEA levels decrease after age 30, and are reported low in critically ill people.)

CALORIE RESTRICTION

Tests on mice and fruit flies have proven that semi-starvation does extend life . . . up to 40 percent. There is now evidence that calorie restriction works in primates and humans, too, which has made the idea of the Calorie Restriction Diet a popular way to increase longevity.

More than twenty years ago, two groups of rhesus monkeys were studied. One group was placed on a calorie-restricted diet. Last year, researchers reported how the monkeys on diets were healthier with less diabetes, cancer, and heart disease. Even their brains were younger. "These data demonstrate that caloric restriction slows aging in a primate species," reported Ricki J. Colman and Richard Weindruch (*New York Times*, July 9, 2009). Weindruch and David Allison, a statistician, expect the dieting monkeys will live 10 to 20 percent longer, which is promising for humans. These monkeys and mice started their diets when they were somewhere between six and fourteen years old, but mice placed on restricted diets from birth demonstrated the most striking life span extensions.

A longevity diet developed by the late UCLA professor and author of *Beyond the 120 Year Diet, Maximum Lifespan and the Anti-Aging Plan*, Roy Walford, uses a combination of Calorie Restriction with Optimum Nutrition (CRON) to reduce calorie intake with eating the right amounts of nutrients (like protein, fat, carbohydrates, vitamins, minerals, fiber, and probiotic bacteria) to help maintain a healthy body, desired levels of activity, and extend life.

Walford found that "the calorically restricted low-fat nutrient-dense diet . . . significantly lowers blood glucose, total leukocyte count, cholesterol, and blood pressure in humans" (*Proceedings of the National Academy of Sciences*, Dec. 1992).

The first studies on calorie restriction were reported in 1935; studies continue to show that CR extends life spans and increases longevity for species including yeasts, worms, mice, and as recent studies indicate, primates . Molecular studies have shown that some genes create enzymes increasing mitochondrial activity, and slow the cell's aging processes (H. Yang et al., "Nutrient-Sensitive Mitochondrial NAD+ Levels Dictate Cell Survival," *Cell*, Volume 130, no. 5, Sept. 21, 2007).

One important thing to note is that it's easier to develop nutritional deficiencies while on a calorie-restricted diet, especially if the diet doesn't include a wide range of food to provide trace nutrients. Since raw foods can be a lower calorie diet, it is important to ensure we get a wide spectrum of nutrients from a broad array of different fruits, vegetables, nuts, and seeds to keep healthy.

WHEN TO EAT

One of the leading theories of aging is the glycemic theory, which says excess glucose leads to pathological changes. Grazing and eating smaller meals throughout the day prevents glucose from rising excessively after eating. Whereas eating a lot of food at once has been shown to elevate blood glucose levels. Increasing the amount of fiber will slow the absorption of carbohydrates and sugar. Some calorie restriction people will consume about 60 percent of their calories from fat and a small number from carbohydrates to avoid eating large quantities of food at one time.

Eating smaller snacks throughout the day also is beneficial in weight loss and boosting of our metabolism. Think of our metabolism as a fire. We want this fire to burn constantly through the day, so we need to keep stoking it by adding a log on every few hours. Put too many logs on at once, and you risk putting the fire out. A trainer once told me to eat a small bowlful of food only when I got hungry, the small bowl being equivalent to the size of both my palms. Eating this volume, I found I was hungry every 2–3 hours or so without having to time my snacks.

WHAT TO EAT

Our U.S. Recommended Daily Allowance of 2,000 calories a day, used as reference in nutrition labels, is made up of 15 percent protein, 30 percent fat, and 55 percent carbohydrates. The high carbohydrate content has been blamed for the obesity issues in the United States. Calorie restricted diets include nutrient rich, low calorie foods to provide 30 percent protein, 30 percent fat, and 40 percent carbohydrates. In raw food, this simply translates into sea vegetables, greens, wheatgrass, nuts, seeds, and fruit.

The Glycemic Index, or GI, was developed about twenty years ago for diabetics to encourage eating more complex carbohydrates that digest and process slower than simple sugars. A food's GI level is ranked on a scale from 1 to 100, and measures blood glucose levels over 2 hours after a food's eaten. A score of 0 to 55 is low, 56 to 69 medium, and 70 to 100 high glycemic. Low-GI foods help avoid spikes and sharp declines in blood glucose, for a steadier stream of energy, and help us avoid damage to our arteries and blood vessels while reducing the risk of heart disease.

Spikes in glucose levels and insulin caused by high GI diet means too much insulin is in our body, which causes us to store fat and makes it harder to burn it off. High-GI foods also make us more hungry, especially when the glucose drops and the crash happens. Low-GI foods keep us fuller longer.

Jennie Brand-Miller, coauthor of *The Low GI Handbook*, says to eat fruits and vegetables, except potatoes, daily, and she recommends filling half your plate with fruits and vegetables, one quarter with protein, and one quarter with low-GI carbohydrate. Keep in mind that vegetables contain low GI carbs.

IDEAL WEIGHT

It's been documented that obesity increases likelihood of life-shortening diseases like diabetes, cancer, heat disease. But the actual body mass index for longevity and mental health is still to be proven. What's been shown in people who have lived over a hundred years is that they stayed their same weight as they aged. Since our metabolism does slow with aging, this means decreasing the number of calories we eat as we age. Exercise and lean muscle mass will also keep our metabolism from slowing down as much, and helps maintain consistent body weight.

WELLNESS

Wellness is an equation taking aspects of our mind, body, and spirit into account. Meditation, rest, fitness, rejuvenation exercises like yoga or taichi, being part of a community, our outlook on life, and positive thinking together contribute to longevity, even when body mass is higher. It's a combination of more than just diet, it's our overall lifestyle and level of happiness.

Things I've Learned

For me, life is about always being curious, learning, and expanding my view of our world while continuing to challenge myself to push boundaries and grow.

I used to feel so righteous in the way I was living. My life became narrow, focused, and very controlled. One day I made a decision to open up my world to extend beyond my narrow path. I longed to experience things as if for the first time again, and I wanted to be open to inspiration from outside my narrow bubble. I also remembered where I came from. I was a Korean American shaped by my experiences of growing up Asian in America.

The most profound change came during my first visit to Singapore, Bali, and Thailand in late 2009. For the first time in my life, I experienced what it felt like to fit in, to be treated as a local. Even on my previous trips to Korea, I've stood out. I was bigger and taller, dressed in different clothing, and carried myself differently. But in South East Asia, where it's a mix of different Asians of various sizes, shades of color, straight and curly hair, I fit in. When I returned to America, everything looked different to me. It was suddenly clear that who I am, how I think, and how I act has been shaped by my cultural background as an Asian American. And this is what's inspired me to write this book.

I hope to share with you some clarity I've gained along my journey toward health and longevity. I'm finally discovering the importance of balance and grounding.

A LIFE OUT OF BALANCE

Raw foods helped me undo much of the damage from my earlier years of partying and putting less than healthy things into my body. I felt vibrant, healthy, had tons of energy and enthusiasm, and felt like I could take on the world. The mental clarity, focus, and energy raw foods gave me enabled me to put tons of energy into building my first raw food business, SmartMonkey Foods.

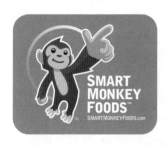

What began as an events and catering company in the late '90s quickly expanded into a line of prepared packaged foods, workshops, classes, retreats, a weekly café, catering, and then a line of fruit and nut bars available across all of Canada and in most major U.S. markets. Raw foods fueled me to work long hours juggling many roles in the office all day. Many times, I would also work in the evenings and sometimes through the night at our commercial kitchen when employees called in sick.

By 2006, the business had grown very large, and my partner Ede Schweizer and I needed more help. We brought in a friend of mine who I'd known for over a decade as a third partner. Around the same time, Ede and I decided to part ways. The very next day, Ede was offered an amazing career opportunity in California and I was given my first cookbook deal. It was as if the universe agreed Ede and I would affect more change by spreading our circles of influence separately, rather than together as one.

I wanted to return to California, but first needed to sell my house in Portland, Oregon. In short, due to permits and renovations, it took nearly a year for the house to sell. On top of that, I was on my own for the first time in over seven years, the manuscript for my first book, *Ani's Raw Food Kitchen*, was due in a few months, and SmartMonkey Foods was busier than ever. I was completely overwhelmed.

Looking back today, I can say this final year in Portland was the most stressful year of my life, and I was living completely out of balance. I was eating raw foods, but too much cacao and sweet fruits, and was too busy to properly balance my nutritional intake. I was also suffering from extreme insomnia, sleeping only an hour a night because my brain refused to stop thinking. In an attempt to exhaust myself, I would exercise super hard for 2 to 3 hours. I'd fight sleep all day in an attempt to sleep better at night, and I'd be out like a light when it was time for bed. The crazy thing is that I'd awake an hour later energized and ready to start my day. I'd get up and work all night long. The sun would eventually come up, and the vicious cycle of unrest, stress, and anxiety would repeat all over again.

It's hardly surprising that this lack of rest, extreme exercise, stress, and worry threw off the balance in my body. Compounded by my previous fifteen-plus years of living out of balance and working too hard, it finally manifested on the physical level as vertigo. Looking back now, it makes logical sense how a lack of balance in mind, body, and spirit would create the inability to balance physically. I continued to have vertigo episodes that lasted two to three days every three months for over two years. These bouts were fully debilitating. Without balance, I couldn't sit up, stand, walk, and could only lie still in bed with my eyes closed. Moving would start my head spinning and I'd feel nauseous. It was terrible and extremely frightening.

TAKING MY CLIMATE INTO CONSIDERATION

An integrative medicine doctor who had taught me so much about raw food nutrition, cleansing, and detoxing many years prior had started to tell me for a couple of years that I needed to reintroduce cooked foods like quinoa and fish into my diet. He could tell by looking at me that I was out of balance and suffering from deficiencies. Other health practitioners would feel my freezing cold hands and tell me pretty much the same thing. "Raw foods may work well in hot climates, but not so well in the cold and damp Pacific Northwest," and "Take an orchid out of the rainforest, put it in the Arctic, and it will die." I refused to listen to anyone, and continued to add "heat" to my foods with spicy chile, garlic, and ginger.

In October 2006, I visited my family in Korea for the first time in over 17 years. My aunt took one look at me and was convinced she needed to take me to Shanghai to the Chinese Medical Research Center to see a doctor, and immediately began booking our travel plans. While in Korea, I was taken to another Korean doctor versed in Ayurveda, Chinese, and Korean medicine. Both doctors came to the same conclusion. I had dampness in my kidneys, and my internal fire, or Chi, had been extinguished by eating cold damp raw foods in a cold, damp environment. I desperately needed to get my flame burning again.

The Korean doctor told me to eat freshwater fish along with produce that grows in water (like sea vegetables), in the ground, or in the shade (like broccoli, cauliflower, beets, radishes, kale). He explained that vegetables that grow in water or low light do so because they naturally contain an excess of heat. Sea vegetables were good for stoking my internal fire because they are so hot they need to grow in cold water. On the other hand, cucumbers are known for their cooling property, and grow in bright sunlight. So do peppers and tomatoes. I was to avoid cold produce that grows in the hot sun. This made logical sense to me.

After I returned back to Portland, I started a course of Chinese herbs and acupuncture. It was November, cold, and rainy in Portland. I finally decided to listen to what all the doctors had been telling me. I began introducing more cooked and warming foods like quinoa, garbanzo beans, lentils, and sweet potatoes into my diet. After I discovered sensitivity to wheat and soy, I stuck with legumes, quinoa, and occasional steamed vegetables. Fearful of vertigo, and desperate to avoid another episode, I even tried eating fish. And in time, this path healed me.

LAYING ROOTS TO BALANCE

Today, I'm grateful to have restored my health. As I look back, it's clear to me how extreme I was living. Even after I finally sold my home in December 2006 and left Oregon, I gave away and sold almost all of my possessions as a spiritual and emotional cleanse. I lived on the road without a home base for over a year. Kanga my pooch rode with me in my Mercedes 560 SL, and everything we owned fit into the trunk of my tiny coupe. This new freedom was liberating after being bound to my huge home for a year longer than I'd desired. I liked how not having a solid home base forced me to remain open and flexible. I was now fully open and inviting of new energy and opportunities to flow into my life.

It wasn't until I had discovered Vipassana meditation, which I'll explain later, and laid down my roots in West Hollywood in early 2009 that my vertigo spells ended. The prior 3 years had been unbalanced and challenging; when I found Vipassana, I found my footing again. As soon as I made the decision to be still, grounded, to call this place home, and to lay down my roots, everything seemed to stabilize at all levels of my mind, body, and spirit.

STRESS

Stress activates our "flight or flight" response, which is considered to be a good thing in the right situations. Back in the days when we were living in caves, predators would trigger our fight or flight response in our brains' limbic system. It's hardwired into our bodies. This response mechanism is what boosts our defense against infections and traumas like cuts and bruises. However, on the other hand, long-term stress that causes anxiety is bad for our overall health and immune system.

I strive to decrease all types of stressors including environmental stress that comes in via toxins in the air I breathe and the water I shower in, to the emotional anxiety of everyday life, to physical stress due to a lack of rest, to nutritional stress placed on my body from unhealthy foods that are hard to digest, and by taxing myself by exercising too much. By letting go of my expectations when things become a struggle, forgiving myself and others, making time for myself to play, meditating, spending time with loved ones, volunteering and giving back to my community, and laughing as much as possible, I strive to live a Super Life.

AGE AND WISDOM

On my last visit to Korea, my seventy-five-year-old retired uncle got dressed formally in a nice suit. A limousine was outside waiting to drive him back to the science research center he had been the director of for several decades prior. He was being called back to share his wisdom and knowledge that only comes with age. This reminded me of how in Asia, unlike in America, age and wisdom is highly regarded, respected, and revered. And, more than money, education and knowledge is valued.

In America, we fight to hold on to our youth, even if it means risking our lives or making ourselves very sick through excessive dieting and plastic surgery or procedures like Botox. We try to stave off aging in the most unnatural ways. Rather than a notion of aging gracefully, we're obsessed with "anti"-aging. Elders in America are thought of as a nuisance. We are quick to reduce them to childlike status—we throw away their wisdom, and lose everything we have to gain from their hard-won lessons.

DIGNITY, HONOR, RESPECT

To have dignity is to have respect for oneself. To have honor is to be a source of credit and distinction. And to respect denotes a positive feeling of esteem for a person. These values of dignity, honor, and respect for oneself and others are woven throughout Asian culture. The good of the community and group is most important. Harming others to benefit oneself is looked down upon.

I'm hardly perfect, but I do try to remember the giants who came before me, and give credit where credit is due. Without the contributions they made, I would not even have the opportunities that come to me. This is where dignity, respect, and honor play a role. Asian cultures have rituals and ceremonies honoring our ancestors and those who came before us. Asian culture is about the good for the whole, rather than the good of only one person. Thinking this way helps makes it easier to choose the right decisions to avoid harming others.

We don't need to act out of desperation and lack. Realizing our worth and value means we know our chance and time will come.

COMMUNITY

I grew up in a household with an ill father who would eventually pass on to the next level. Dad, like many Koreans of his generation, had contracted tuberculosis from a contaminated water supply in North Korea when he was younger. The antibiotics used to treat it was so strong it damaged his kidneys.

It's painful to remember how he shouldered his illness alone, rather than seeking community and support. That is a downfall in Asian culture, to save face. It's seen as an embarrassment for others to know anything's wrong because it draws attention to one's self. You don't want to stand out, it's rather about being part of the group.

I watched my mother work hard to raise my brother and me. When I look back now, I'm amazed at how she would stay up all night with my dad when his blood pressure was too high to lay down for fear of falling into a coma. Then, she'd go to work all day without a wink of sleep. Mom would drive my dad two hours or more to the hospital, come back, take care of Max and me, and then go back to work. She put us through an Ivy league university on her pharmacist salary. She was in survival mode all those years, with little time for friends and community, compounded with the struggle of English as a second language in small mountain towns that were primarily, if not all, Caucasian.

Mom always encouraged me to study and work hard, to save money, and be successful. I realize now why it was so important that I be financially secure. She didn't want me to struggle as she did. In the mid-'90s, I had an opportunity to work on an Internet project with Miramax to bring streaming films online. My family had planned our vacation and had booked a house in Puerto Vallarta, Mexico. But mom canceled it all so I could work instead. Work always came first. And, this is still a habit I strive to tame.

Mom's changed her tune now, especially since she's retired. It makes me happy to hear of her lunches with college girlfriends, dinners with old colleagues, and trips to Las Vegas with elementary school girlfriends. She's started to tell me to stop working so much because I'm successful enough, which is sweet to hear. She's always encouraging me to fall in love and to enjoy life.

There's a base financial threshold that, when met, one can move away from living in survival mode to enjoy more of the "nice to haves" like fitness, travel, time to take better care of ourselves, a bigger house, and a newer car. Anything above and beyond this minimum threshold is excess and not necessary for mere survival. Native tribes in America worked only about 3 hours a day, as do natives of Bali, to secure food and shelter. Rather than amassing more possessions, the rest of their day is spent creating arts and crafts, enjoying family and friends, making and sharing good food, and laughing.

Over the past decade or more, key leaders in our raw food movement have worked hard to create successful businesses. Lately, several have told me they are feeling isolated and alone after years of focusing and pushing hard to create our new paradigm. A cure for feeling disconnected is to come together to share our gifts. In this way, our movement will become larger and will make an even bigger impression on the world. Besides, I find it to be much more fun to work in partnership with others than by myself in isolation.

GIVING BACK

In the past few years what I've been enjoying most is teaching and working with children, especially underprivileged and at-risk youth living in lower-income areas. Most of these neighborhoods are nutritional deserts—they don't have real food available in their markets. All that's available are processed and packaged nonfoods like brightly colored orange cheese puffs or mac and cheese out of a dusty box. There are inequalities and systemic barriers making sustainable communities and self-reliant lifestyles unattainable for people in these communities.

Parents in these areas usually work two to three jobs, struggling to make ends meet. They have little money, no time, and few options for preparing healthy food for their families. Kids are overweight and obese and many are on the road to developing Type 2 diabetes. A sustainable local food system where food is grown, distributed, and purchased within the community, paired with training and educational programs, is needed in these, and all, communities. The creation of jobs and partnerships with regional farmers would benefit these communities, too.

Teaching children how to grow food helps boosts self-confidence and self-reliance. Gardening connects kids to the earth and life, and helps them understand where food comes from. All kids love to care for and to watch plants grow.

The next step is to teach these kids how to use the produce from their garden to make healthy delicious food. This way, they can take this skill into their homes and make food to share with their families from the ground up. In time, this will spread to create positive change across the whole community. When these kids have the power to grow their own food, become connected to life, and begin to fuel their bodies and brains with real nutrients from the earth, they'll feel great and do amazing things. To give back, to create change, to help make lives better for kids is what most excites my soul these days.

MEDITATION

I was on a quest to find balance and discovered Vipassana, which is not a religion; but rather, is a style of meditation the Buddha spent the rest of his life teaching after reaching enlightenment. Vipassana helped to put the world into perspective for me. When I left Portland, I realized I had already started to practice non-attachment by letting go of all my physical possessions, and even my home. Now, it was time to work on letting go of my emotional and mental cravings for things that felt good and my aversion away from things that felt bad. I learned that there is no "good" or "bad." Things just are what they are. Vipassana reminded me how at the quantum physics level, we are not solid, but vibration. I believe raw foods play a part in setting the frequency at which I resonate. And I could feel this vibration when I sat still.

I had tried many styles of meditation and attended numerous workshops to learn to sit still, but it never snapped into place until I discovered Vipassana. I embarked on a silent 10-day program tucked away in the mountains near Yosemite National Park in central California. No phones, computers, paper, books, pens . . . nothing was allowed to distract us from the task at hand, learning to mediate.

Delicious vegetarian and mostly vegan foods were prepared and served for us by volunteers. These volunteers were practicing being in service to help another person have this truly life changing experience. I didn't need to worry about a thing, everything was provided for. Every time my mind would grow restless, the fact of the matter was, there was nowhere for me to go and nothing for me to do, except sit and meditate.

It's challenging to wake at 4 a.m. to start mediating through to 9 p.m., with breaks for meals and stretching. The first few days were hard. My body ached all over. Finally, it all clicked for me on day 5. I got to a place where time flew by. I could suddenly easily sit still for an hour or more. It was in this moment I realized how our minds create chatter and distraction. While sitting in meditation, a sharp pain would appear in my leg or back. But as soon as we could move at the end of the hour, the pain instantly disappeared. This perception of pain was just my mind trying to distract me from the task at hand.

Vipassana meditators follow precepts including abstaining from killing any being or causing stress to any other living being, along with abstaining from stealing, telling lies, and using intoxicants. These philosophies flow into how one chooses to live, and even the careers we choose. We must not choose a job that harms others, like building missiles or selling firearms. Instead, it's important to earn a noble living without having to cheat, steal, lie, or create harm to other living beings. In Thailand, India, and other parts of Southeast Asia, Vipassana is a way of life. It permeates everything throughout the day. You can see it in the way people treat one another, in the diet, and how people handle things throughout the day.

May we all thrive, rather than merely survive, by being more compassionate, honest, healthy, respectful, and considerate. Let's all feel more passionate, happy, and alive. Go Super Life!

MY RAW FOOD SHAPE-SHIFTING

As I began enjoying more fresh, local, organic, seasonal produce, I immediately noticed changes in my physical, mental, emotional, and spiritual self. Raw foods affected my environment, too.

ENERGY

After my first gourmet raw meal, I was awake all night long effortlessly preparing for a presentation early the next morning. The presentation went off without a hitch, even without much sleep. The next day, I felt good and discovered I could function well on very little rest with the help of raw food, which is not always a good thing. Prolonged lack of rest can cause imbalances in one's system, which I learned the hard way years later. I remember how friends would tease me because I was using raw foods like speed, the drug, to sleep less and get tons done at work and at play. Raw foods gave me a new level of mental clarity and focus. I was hyper-productive, could multitask like crazy, and on many days would complete the work of three people at one time.

I felt strong, energetic, and powerful. My stamina and endurance seemed to increase even when I didn't work out as much. And, I lost 15 pounds in the first month of stuffing myself full of gourmet raw foods. An athlete my entire life, I didn't realize I had 15 pounds to lose. And, I desperately needed cleansing and detoxing at the physical level from over a decade of partying, drinking, and dancing all night long during the rave years in London, Sydney, and San Francisco.

EMOTIONS

On the emotional level, I felt even more compassion toward all living beings. I was more level-headed, felt less toxic, and was less erratically emotional. I contribute this partially to the fact that once I began eating cleaner, my body felt better and fueled my happiness. When I'm happy, it's much easier to let things bounce off me than when I'm not feeling so good. I'm an emotional being, and raw foods helped make the range between my peaks and valleys shallower. I continue to strive to find the right balance, that's my lifelong pursuit.

>>>

>>>

SPIRITUALITY

I am intrigued by the ideas of quantum physics. It says that people and everything around us are all made up of vibrations, and nothing is solid state. That means each of us vibrates at a different frequency. It makes sense to think that different people can hum and purr together creating a beautiful melody, while others clash like flat keys on a piano.

When I discovered Raw Foods 2.0 (what I define as the gourmet cuisine of today, rather than the Raw Food 1.0 I was raised on), I initially found I became more judgmental, believing I'd stumbled upon the one and only way for everyone to eat and live. Raw foods can seem like a cult in that way. I'm happy I woke up to later realize this extreme outlook creates barriers rather than invitations for others to join me in my quest for optimal health, happiness, and longevity.

I discovered anything in extremes is unhealthy. My extreme outlook on living a perfect vegan and raw-food lifestyle added a level of stress to my life. And the effects of this stress were compounded over time. I've always loved animals, and now I felt an even stronger level of compassion for them and all living beings. I believe being connected to the earth through our food gives us a sense of connectedness to all life.

ENVIRONMENT

On an environmental level, I noticed an immediate drop in the amount of garbage my home produced. Since my produce, nuts, and seeds now came from farmers' markets and in bulk quantities, I no longer found prepared food packaging in my trash bins. Instead, what I had left was organic compost, which creates new life, and some recyclables.

I began saving glass jars and containers to use for storing leftovers, nuts, seeds, and spices. I became more sensitive and aware of toxic chemicals in my environment like household and industrial cleansers, personal care products, and even polluted air and water. I stopped buying paper towels and napkins, and found it to be more economical to cut apart an old t-shirt or to use an old sponge to clean the floors in my house.

I threw away my nail polish and toxic skin care products as soon as I realized how anything I put onto my skin absorbs into my body. And the integrative medicine doctor who taught me how to cleanse through his 21 Day Detox program (www.21daydetox.com) convinced me to stop taking pharmaceuticals including birth control pills. It took eight years for my menstrual cycle to normalize itself. But today, at the age of 42, it's more regular than it ever was.

All of these changes on the physical, mental, emotional, spiritual, and environmental levels contributed to my increased vitality and health, along with a repaired, regenerated, and cleaner body. Over the years, I've watched my body's needs shift over time. I also discovered the hard way that my extreme lifestyle, beyond just my diet, had caused imbalances to build up in my body.

ACKNOWLEDGMENTS

Thank you Jae Phyo (aka Jaekil Cho), my mother, Inchol Joseph Phyo, my late father, and Max Phyo, my brother, for my wonderful Asian American life and for all the love you pour into it. Thank you for showing me how to appreciate both Western and Eastern cultures and for teaching me how to grow my own food, how to live a toxin-free life, and how to tread lightly on our planet. Mom and Dad, you were both the first eco-green lifestylists I've known.

My aunts Namah Cho (aka Mrs. Joo) and Jaehee Cho (aka Mrs. Park), my cousin Minnie Roh, and SoYoung Lee, thank you for helping me understand and translate traditional Korean recipes. Thank you Dr. Ruben Cartegena for sharing medical, health, and healing wisdom and for taking loving care of mom.

Tyler Golden, thank you and assistant Steven Alders for taking mouthwatering recipe photos once again. Thank you Thea Maichle for making our photo shoots about play. Antonio Sanchez, I'm blessed to have the coolest illustrations in all my books. You're the world's best illustrator. Maria Loewenstein and Arthur Davis III (KingVictoria™), and your team: Pablo Sanchez, Lisa Dempsey, Alex David, and Jaime Padilla, I'm amazed at how you're able to make me look like a model; your positivity is contagious. Anthony Hall, your Asia environmental photos are beautiful and remind me of our journey in Phuket. Marieke Derks, thank you for the Mom Tri's Villa Royale photos, and Sylvie Yaffe, thanks for helping make this happen. My friends Carol Conforti and Chris Synn, thank you for joining me on an adventure of a lifetime in Bali.

Thank you SmartMonkey testers for helping to ensure these recipes are easy to follow and taste yummy: Jae Phyo, John Johnson, Jennifer M. Smith, Grant Nivison, Lyndsay Braswell, and Angela Minelli. A special thank you to my friend and mentor Spencer Christian for sharing extensive wine pairing expertise and for being a huge inspiration in my life.

A very special thanks to Kato Banks, Tina Dubois Wexler, Shadi Azarpour, Renee Sedliar, William F. Ahmann, and Eric Weissler for your continued unwavering support and love. Thank you Da Capo: Kevin Hanover, Kate Kazeniac Burke, Lindsey Triebel, Alex Camlin, and Erica Truxler. It's been so much fun working together over the years. Of course a big thank you to Kanga, my Rhodesian Ridgeback for reminding me to take breaks to stretch, breathe, nap, and love.

Thank YOU, the reader, for taking a peek at my book. I hope this book may inspire you to play in your kitchen more and to have fun whipping up fast tasty treats to share with everyone.

May you feel great, be happy, live long, and Go Super Life!

METRIC CONVERSIONS

- The recipes in this book have not been tested with metric measurements, so some variations might occur.
- Remember that the weight of dry ingredients varies according to the volume or density factor: 1 cup of flour weighs far less than 1 cup of sugar, and 1 tablespoon doesn't necessarily hold 3 teaspoons.

GENERAL FORMULA FOR METRIC CONVERSION

Ounces to grams	ounces × 28.35 = grams
Grams to ounces	grams × 0.035 = ounces
Pounds to grams	pounds × 453.5 = grams
Pounds to kilograms	pounds × 0.45 = kilograms
Cups to liters	cups × 0.24 = liters
Fahrenheit to Celsius	(°F − 32) × 5 ÷ 9 = °C
Celsius to Fahrenheit	(°C × 9) ÷ 5 + 32 = °F

VOLUME (LIQUID) MEASUREMENTS

1 teaspoon = ⅙ fluid ounce = 5 milliliters

1 tablespoon = ½ fluid ounce = 15 milliliters

2 tablespoons = 1 fluid ounce = 30 milliliters

¼ cup = 2 fluid ounces = 60 milliliters

⅓ cup = 2⅔ fluid ounces = 79 milliliters

½ cup = 4 fluid ounces = 118 milliliters

1 cup or ½ pint = 8 fluid ounces = 250 milliliters

2 cups or 1 pint = 16 fluid ounces = 500 milliliters

4 cups or 1 quart = 32 fluid ounces = 1,000 milliliters

1 gallon = 4 liters

OVEN TEMPERATURE EQUIVALENTS, FAHRENHEIT (F) AND CELSIUS (C)

100°F = 38°C

200°F = 95°C

250°F = 120°C

300°F = 150°C

350°F = 180°C

400°F = 205°C

450°F = 230° C

WEIGHT (MASS) MEASUREMENTS

1 ounce = 30 grams

2 ounces = 55 grams

3 ounces = 85 grams

4 ounces = ¼ pound = 125 grams

8 ounces = ½ pound = 240 grams

12 ounces = ¾ pound = 375 grams

16 ounces = 1 pound = 454 grams

VOLUME (DRY) MEASUREMENTS

¼ teaspoon = 1 milliliter

½ teaspoon = 2 milliliters

¾ teaspoon = 4 milliliters

1 teaspoon = 5 milliliters

1 tablespoon = 15 milliliters

¼ cup = 59 milliliters

⅓ cup = 79 milliliters

½ cup = 118 milliliters

⅔ cup = 158 milliliters

¾ cup = 177 milliliters

1 cup = 225 milliliters

4 cups or 1 quart = 1 liter

½ gallon = 2 liters

1 gallon = 4 liters

LINEAR MEASUREMENTS

½ in = 1½ cm

1 inch = 2½ cm

6 inches = 15 cm

8 inches = 20 cm

10 inches = 25 cm

12 inches = 30 cm

20 inches = 50 cm

RESOURCES

Here are more resources and Web sites to help you go—or stay—raw. Included are my e-store, where you'll find my favorite tools and organic ingredients, my Web site with healthy recipes, my uncooking videos, and how to connect with me online. Plus, Web sites where you can find more information on well-being, longevity, meditation, and even safety information on household products. Even my pooch, Kanga, loves raw foods, so I list the recipes I enjoy sharing with her.

KANGA LOVES RAW FOOD

My friends tell me that my dog, Kanga, eats better than they do. Well, everything she eats is the same as what I eat. Preferably local, seasonal, organic when possible, minus common allergens like peanuts, soy, dairy, and wheat. Kanga's my compost bin, eating up all my leftovers and the ends of my carrots, zucchini, and herbs. Crunch is always good for her teeth, and she loves Lotus Root Chips when dehydrated rock hard. Kanga loves durian as much as I do, though we both attempt to eat it in moderation, as with everything. Together, we strive to find a happy balance. Here are some of the recipes your pooch will love you for sharing:

- Nut and Seed Mylk, page 44
- Avocado Shake, minus the Chocolate Sauce, page 51. Kanga loves avocado, but my vet told me that dogs should only eat it on occasion.

- All salads and dressings, but avoid chile spice. Kanga loves Black and Tan Encrusted Coconut Meat, page 78.
- Vegetable Tempura, page 118
- Lotus Root Chips, avoid chile spice, dehydrate completely until rock hard, page 124
- Samosas, page 168
- Corn Fritters, page 176
- Sea vegetables, all, dried. Kanga especially goes nuts for sheets of nori. The texture makes it a fun food for her.

WEBSITES

My websites:

Organic ingredients, superfoods, my favorite kitchen tools (like blenders, dehydrators, ceramic knives, and spiralizers), books and DVDs, and goodies for pets:

- www.GoSuperLife.com

My recipes, cooking videos, eco lifestyle tips, news, and event information:

- www.AniPhyo.com
- www.SmartMonkeyFoods.com

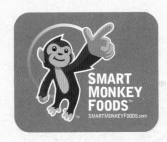

Watch my online videos:

- www.youtube.com/aniphyo

Join me on my social networks:

- www.facebook.com/Ani.Phyo.RawFood
- http://twitter.com/aniphyo

WELL-BEING AND LONGEVITY

Vipassana Meditation

- http://www.dhamma.org/

Happy Planet Index survey, take it and see how happy you are, and at what price to the environment. You may be surprised, I was:

- http://survey.happyplanetindex.org/

Longevity interview on CNN:

- http://us.cnn.com/video/?/video/ international/2009/11/30/vs.clinic .immortality.cnn

Glycemic Index

- www.glycemicindex.com
- www.ginews.blogspot.com

de Grey's vision of human regenerative engineering:

- www.sens.org/

Calorie Restriction Diet (CR):

- www.scientificpsychic.com/health /crondiet.html
- www.crsociety.org/

CRON-O-Meter for tracking nutrients in your foods:

- http://spaz.ca/cronometer/

Why to avoid microwaves:

- www.mercola.com/article/microwave /hazards.htm

Health and safety information on household products:

- http://hpd.nlm.nih.gov/

"Cradle to Cradle," remaking the way we make things:

- www.mcdonough.com/cradle_to _cradle.htm

We are the only species on the planet that creates garbage and landfills. William McDonough and Michael Braungart promote design where waste becomes food for the biosphere so that production and consumption become beneficial for the planet.

- http://video.google.com/videoplay?doc id=-3058533428492266222#
- "Waste = Food" documentary on Cradle to Cradle design concept.

INDEX

CLOSING

If you practice patience, you become more patient.

If you become more patient, you become quieter.

If you become quieter, you become more aware.

If you become more aware, you become more compassionate.

If you become more compassionate, you become more understanding.

If you become more understanding, you become wiser.

If you become wiser, you become more accepting.

If you become more accepting, you become more peaceful.

If you become more peaceful, you will see unity in all things.

If you see unity in all things, you become more grateful.

If you become more grateful, you thank God, you will praise God.

If you praise God, you have understood Life, and the meaning of your life.

And you have come to know that the kingdom of Heaven is indeed within.

—*M. R. Bawa Muhaiyaddeen*

Though I may have felt lost living in a no man's land somewhere between Asia and America for most of my life, today I realize this is the place to be. This space enables a great vantage point for piecing together all the best the East and the West have to offer us.

This blending together of ancient wisdom with the new technologies, the feminine and masculine that creates our whole, and the Yin and the Yang that helps me find the sweet spot for all things Super.

May your life overflow with inner peace, happiness, prosperity, health, wealth, compassion, and love. May it shine brightly onto every being around us, we are all one. Choose peace, happiness, and joy for they are the secrets to enlightenment. Love one, love all. May all beings be happy. Go Super Life.